WHAT KIND OF
A DOG IS THAT?

NINA LEEN

W·W·Norton & Company·New York

Also by Nina Leen:

WOMEN, HEROES, AND A FROG
LOVE, SUNRISE, AND ELEVATED APES
IMAGES OF SOUND
THE WORLD OF BATS
AND THEN THERE WERE NONE
DOGS OF ALL SIZES
SANDIKINS
TAKING PICTURES
THE BAT
SNAKES
MONKEYS

Copyright © 1979 by Nina Leen
Published simultaneously in Canada by George J. McLeod Limited, Toronto. Printed in the United States of America.

All Rights Reserved

First Edition

Library of Congress Cataloging in Publication Data

Leen, Nina
What kind of a dog is that?

   1. Dogs—Identification. 2. Dog breeds. I. Title.
SF426.L43 1977 636.7'1 78–25990
ISBN 0–393–01206–9
ISBN 0–393–01225–5 pbk.

Layout by the author

1 2 3 4 5 6 7 8 9 0

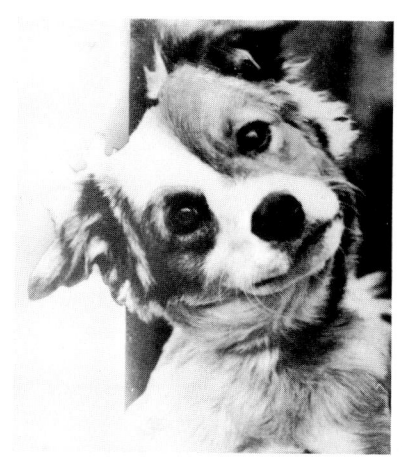

Lucky

Acknowledgments

       I am grateful to David Terry of Quogue, N. Y., for introducing me to his relatives and friends—owners of many appealing mixed-breeds. I wish I could thank every owner and breeder individually, but lack of space makes this impossible.

       I would like to thank Mrs. Marianne Cook, president of the Riverhead Kennel Club, and Dr. Thomas R. Pescod, D.V.M., for their advice and cooperation.

       The Australian Information Service in New York City was very informative and helpful. Also, many thanks to the Time-Life Photo Lab for everything they did to help me. I would like to credit Walter Daran for his picture of the Briard; Robert Grazziano for his picture of the Norwegian Elkhound; and Robert Kelley, © Time Inc., for his picture of the Canadian Husky.

Foreword

There are millions of mixed-breed owners in America; every minute, somewhere in the country, a dog-owner is asked: "What kind of a dog is that?" The answer is usually a slightly embarrassed: "Nothing special...a mongrel." To make the mongrel-owner feel better, he or she is told: "That's the best kind!" I don't agree. All dogs can be true friends, pure-breeds or mixed-breeds, because I am sure that it makes no difference for the owner or the dog what kind each of them is.

Five years ago, I joined the millions of "second-rate" dog-owners—I adopted a stray. Thin, drab-colored, and sparsely furred, she looked like a stray—no question about it. After months of good care, she gained weight, her hair grew long, her colors became bright, and she looked like a possible pure-breed. Since then, on an average of two times a day, I have been asked what kind of a dog she is. Refusing to be humiliated, I considered answers like: "She is half Catalonian Shepherd, half Lapponian Herder..." (both breeds exist), but I soon gave up this idea—I had to find another way to achieve dignity. After all, most pure-breeds evolved after deliberate crossbreeding of dogs with different abilities, dispositions, sizes, and looks—all to produce a dog with necessary qualifications. Common street dogs are in many Champions' ancestry, and many Champions are in the ancestry of today's mongrels. When a dog meets a dog, they don't think of status or family—they mate. Years ago, the usual mix was "Poodle and Cocker Spaniel" or "Shepherd and Collie"; those were the popular breeds in the neighborhoods, and nobody expected his or her dog to meet a Lhasa Apso or a Briard on its daily outings. Then came a change, dogs began to travel, foreign breeds came to this country and every dog had a chance to meet an exotic partner. The offspring of those parents could flaunt a lineage of distinguished ancestors from all parts of the world.

    I found this subject fascinating and started to do some detective work. As a first step, I took pictures of mongrels. As the next step, I interviewed the owners about their dogs. Some of them knew the mother, both parents, and even grandparents of their dogs—but many other owners had never seen the parents; they had to take the word of a previous owner or the animal shelter. Very often the vet made an educated guess.

    If the dog was found or adopted with no information available, I had to find the answers myself. Surrounded by pure-breed dog pictures and countless dog books, I started to study my mixed-breed's pictures, looking for features of pure-breeds reappearing; even a trace could give me a clue to the ancestor. I realized that in many cases, after generations of mongrels, the similarities had been diluted, but I hoped that some features were strong enough to survive in the mongrel descendants.

When I did find "parts" of noble ancestors in faces, coats, tails, and even the characters of the mongrels, there was still no way to know which was a parent, a grandparent, or an ancient forefather—but the important thing was that the ancestors existed and that the mixed-breeds could claim them.

This book was not intended to be a scientific document. I only hope that it can help to diminish the stigma and elevate the self-esteem of the mongrel-owner. When asked the usual question, it's nice to be able to answer: "He is a mix of Basenji and Hovawart!" and have reason to believe it.

N.L.

Pooch looks like the dog "most likely to be adopted." He is a mix of Maltese and Terrier. He can be an angel or a devil—it depends on weather, mood, dinner, and company.

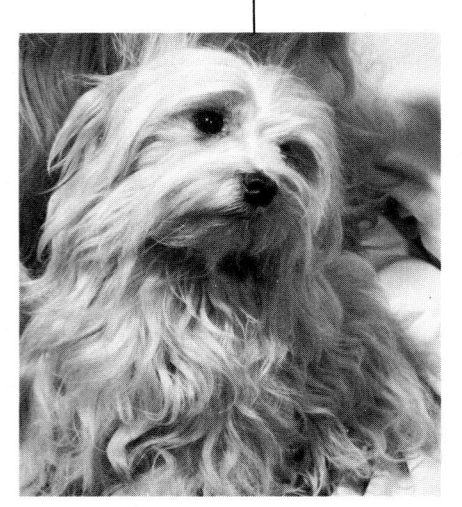

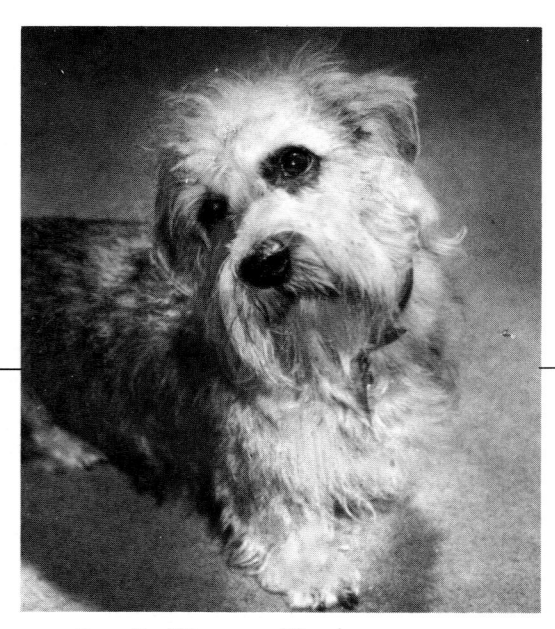

Maltese

Dandie Dinmont Terrier

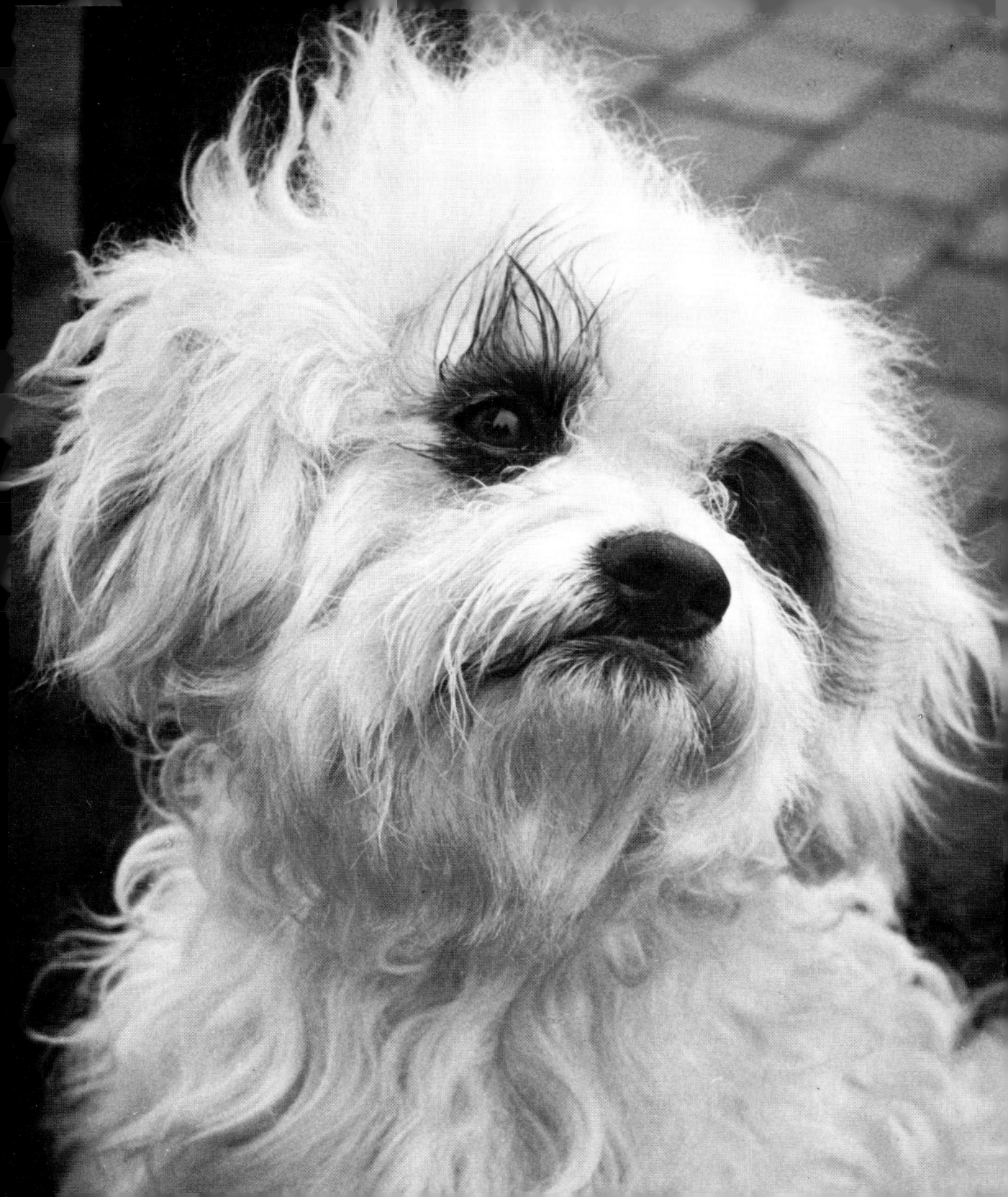

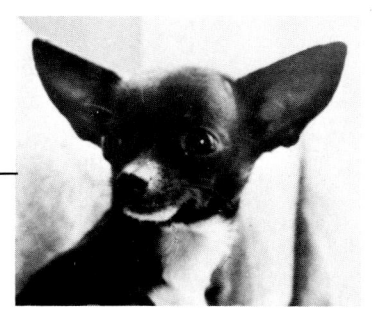

Chihuahua

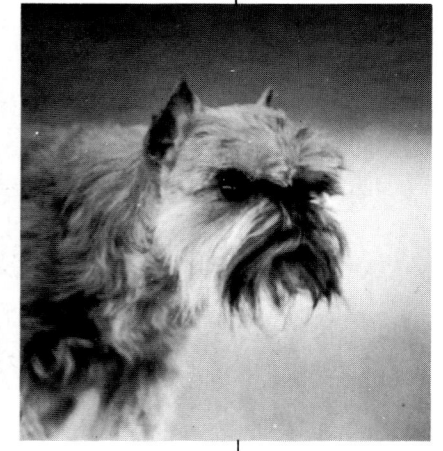

Brussels Griffon

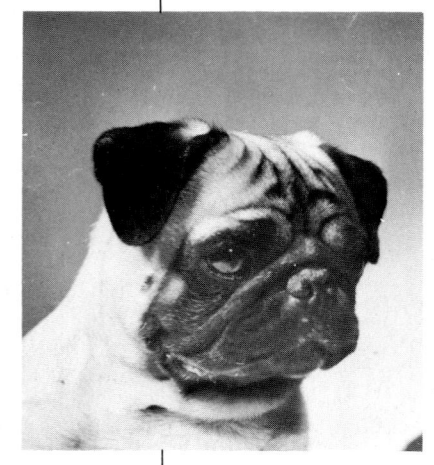

Pug

Affenpinscher

Benny is a small dog,
brimming with self-importance.
His ancestry includes the Pug,
Brussels Griffon, Affenpinscher,
and, according to persistent
rumors, his mother was a Chihuahua.
Nobody knew his father.
He has the loyalty of a Pug, the
temperament of a Griffon, and
the Affenpinscher's terrier blood.
He is a hunter, but instead of
fighting and killing rats as
his ancestors did, he prefers
to chase pheasants. His best
friend is a black-and-white cat.

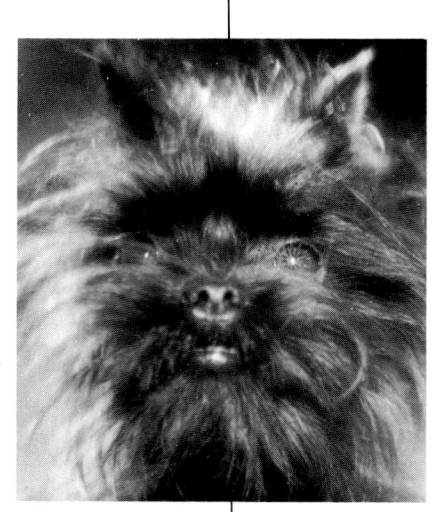

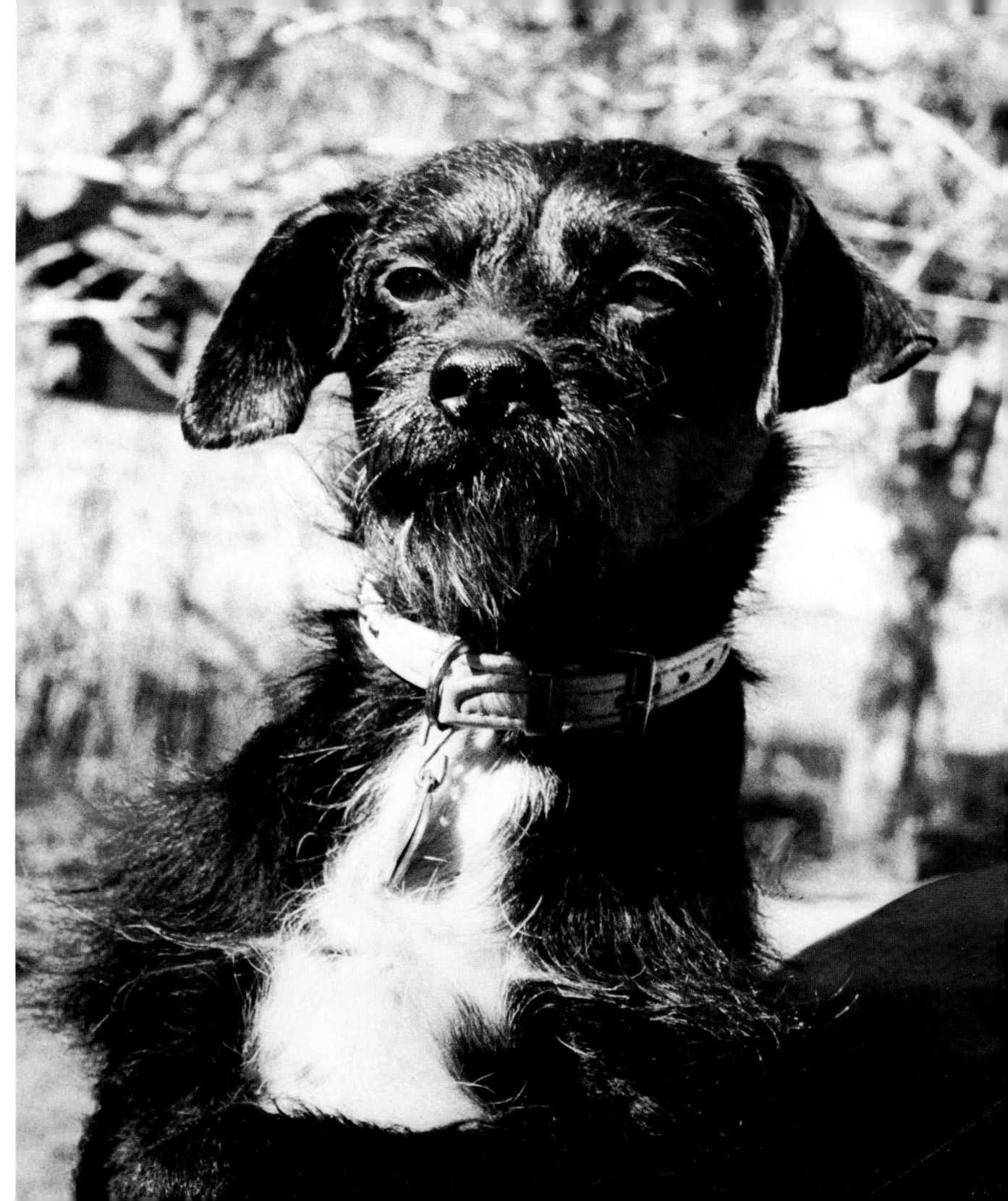

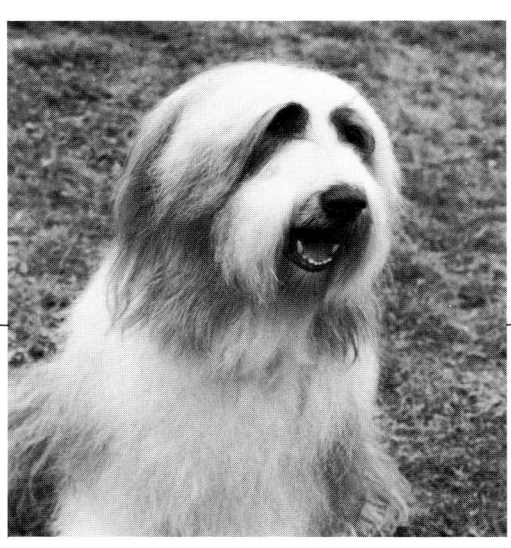

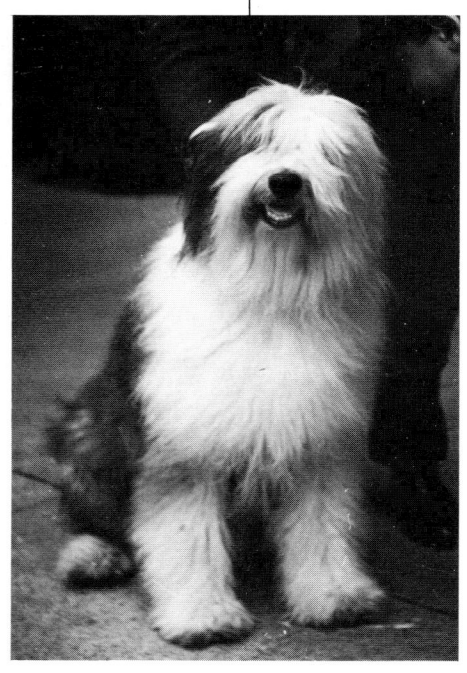

Bearded Collie

Daisy loves the outdoors. Her house is surrounded by woods where she can run and chase squirrels, rabbits, and birds. Even if the hunt is a failure, she enjoys every moment of it. From her ancestors, the Bearded Collie and the Old English Sheepdog, she inherited charm and a much-appreciated weather-resistant coat.

Old English Sheepdog

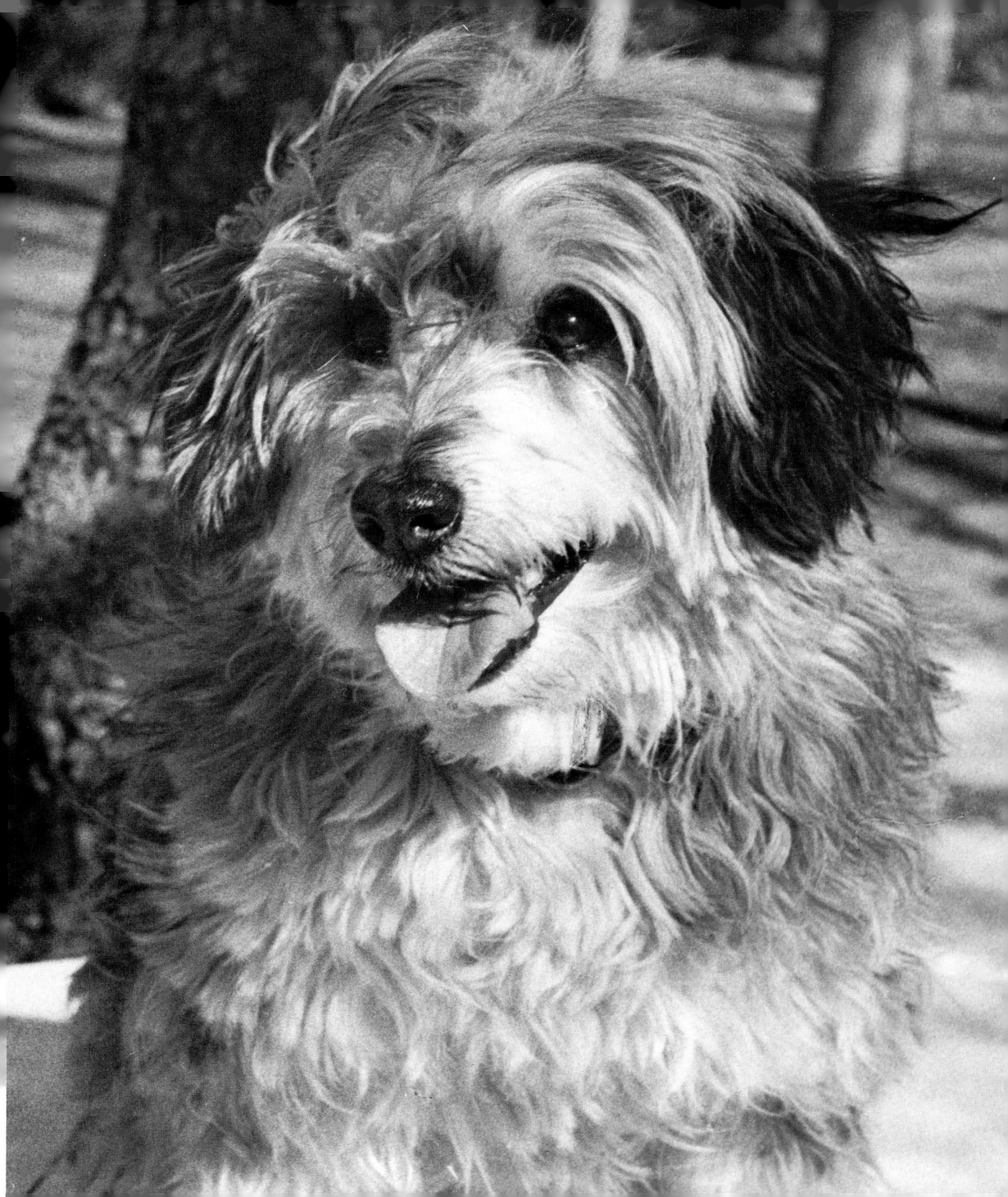

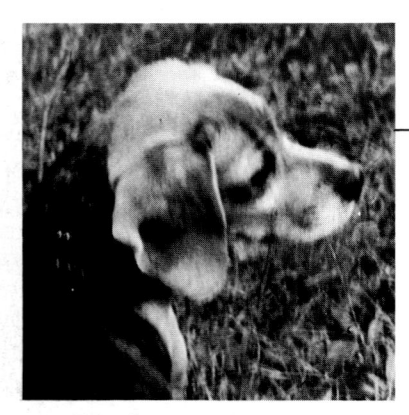

Beagle

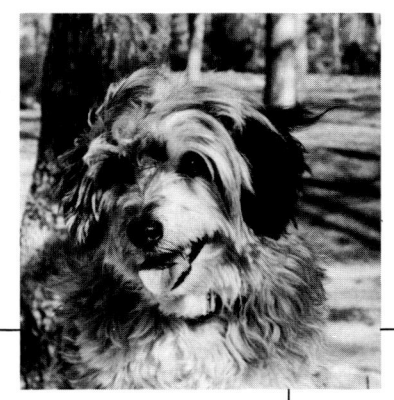

Daisy
Penny's mother

Penny is Daisy's daughter. The father was a Beagle or an Airedale—both were seen in the vicinity of Daisy's woods.
Penny does not live with her mother. She has a nice home, a car, and a big lawn. The only resemblance between Penny and her mother is their winning smile.

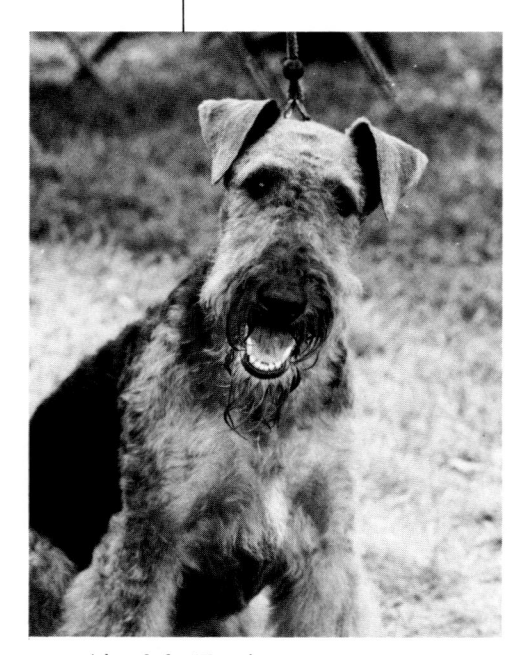

Airedale Terrier

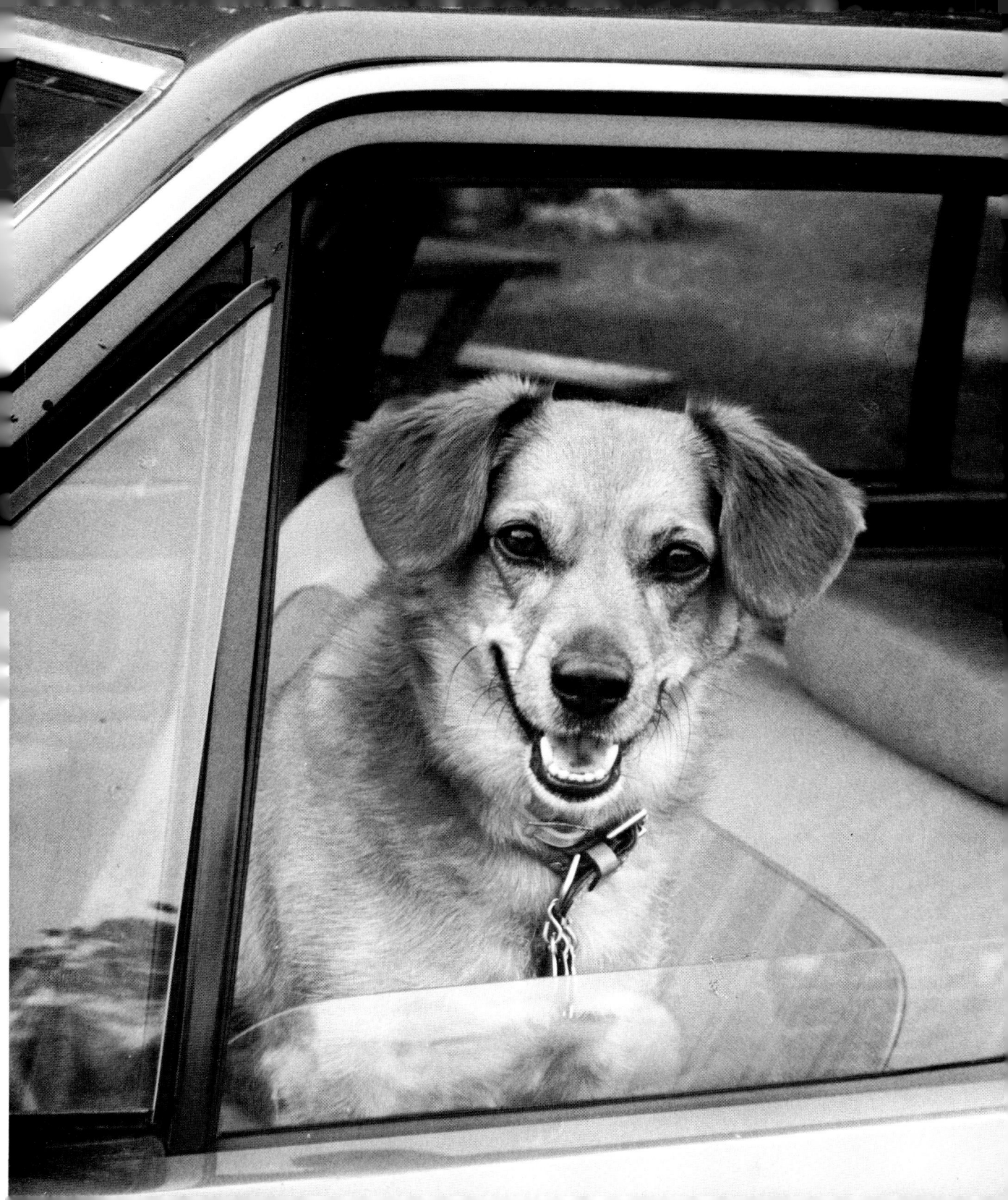

Honey Bear's family came from Alaska. His grandmother Katja, an Alaskan Malamute, has a son, Bear. This son and a Siberian Husky are the parents of Honey Bear. According to native Eskimos, the Alaskan Malamute and the Siberian Husky descended from wolves. Grandmother and father don't show a resemblance to this ancestor, but Honey Bear's similarity to the wolf is obvious. Despite the stern look, Honey Bear is good-natured and "wouldn't hurt a fly."

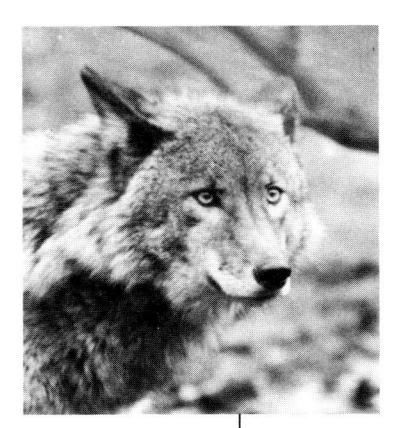

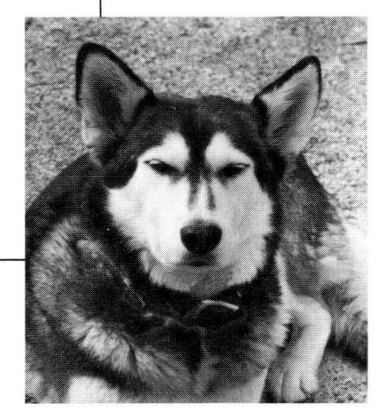

Wolf

Alaskan Malamute
Grandmother, Katja

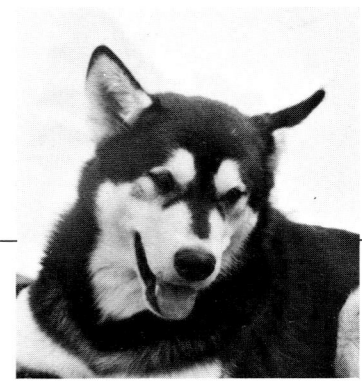

Alaskan Malamute
Father, Bear

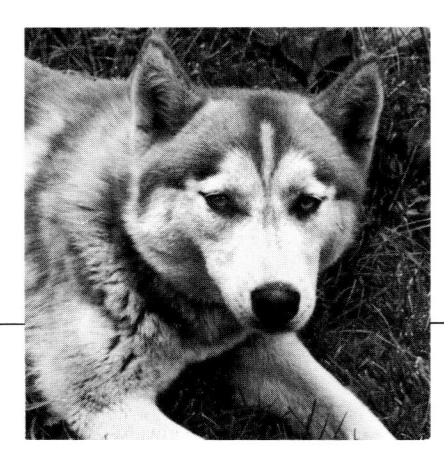

Siberian Husky

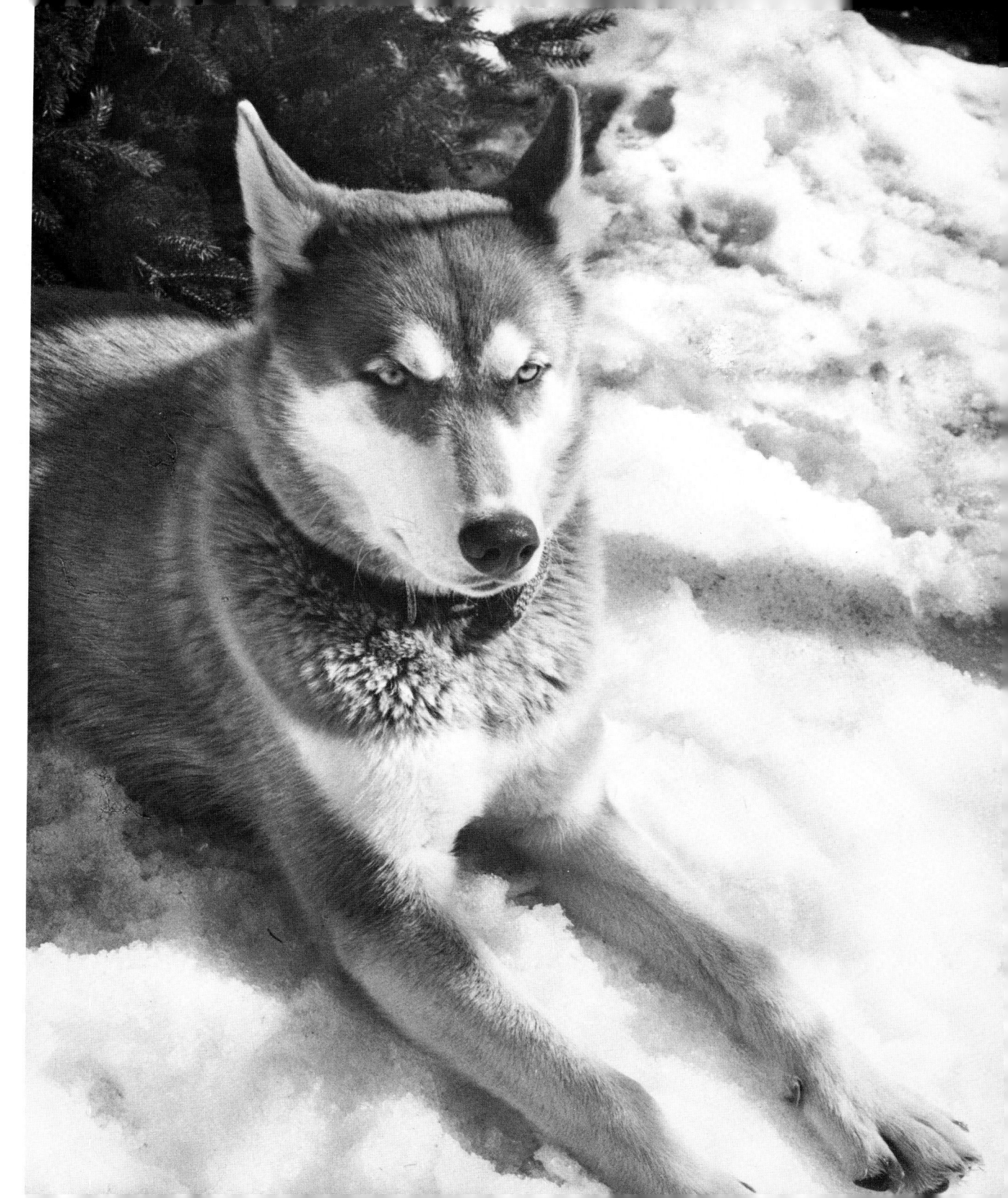

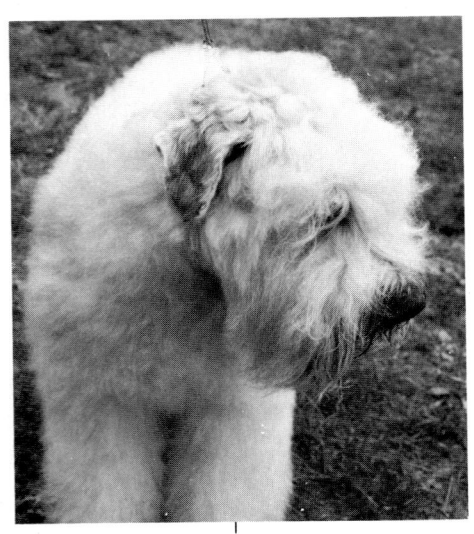

Soft-Coated Wheaten Terrier

Beau is well behaved, never leaves his territory, never goes near cars or strangers. He has the good temper of a Soft-Coated Wheaten Terrier and the winning ways of a Dandie Dinmont Terrier.

But Beau likes to play ball and like all ballplayers is prone to accidents. Making a sharp turn to catch the ball, he tore a ligament in his knee. After days of forced rest the rupture healed and the cast was removed. With gained weight and a new haircut, Beau is ready for the next ballgame.

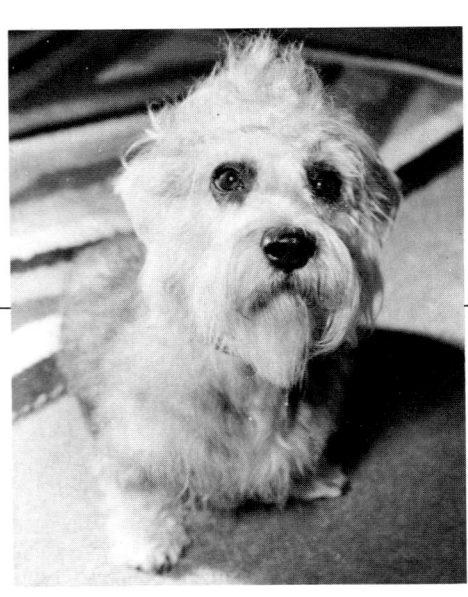

Dandie Dinmont Terrier

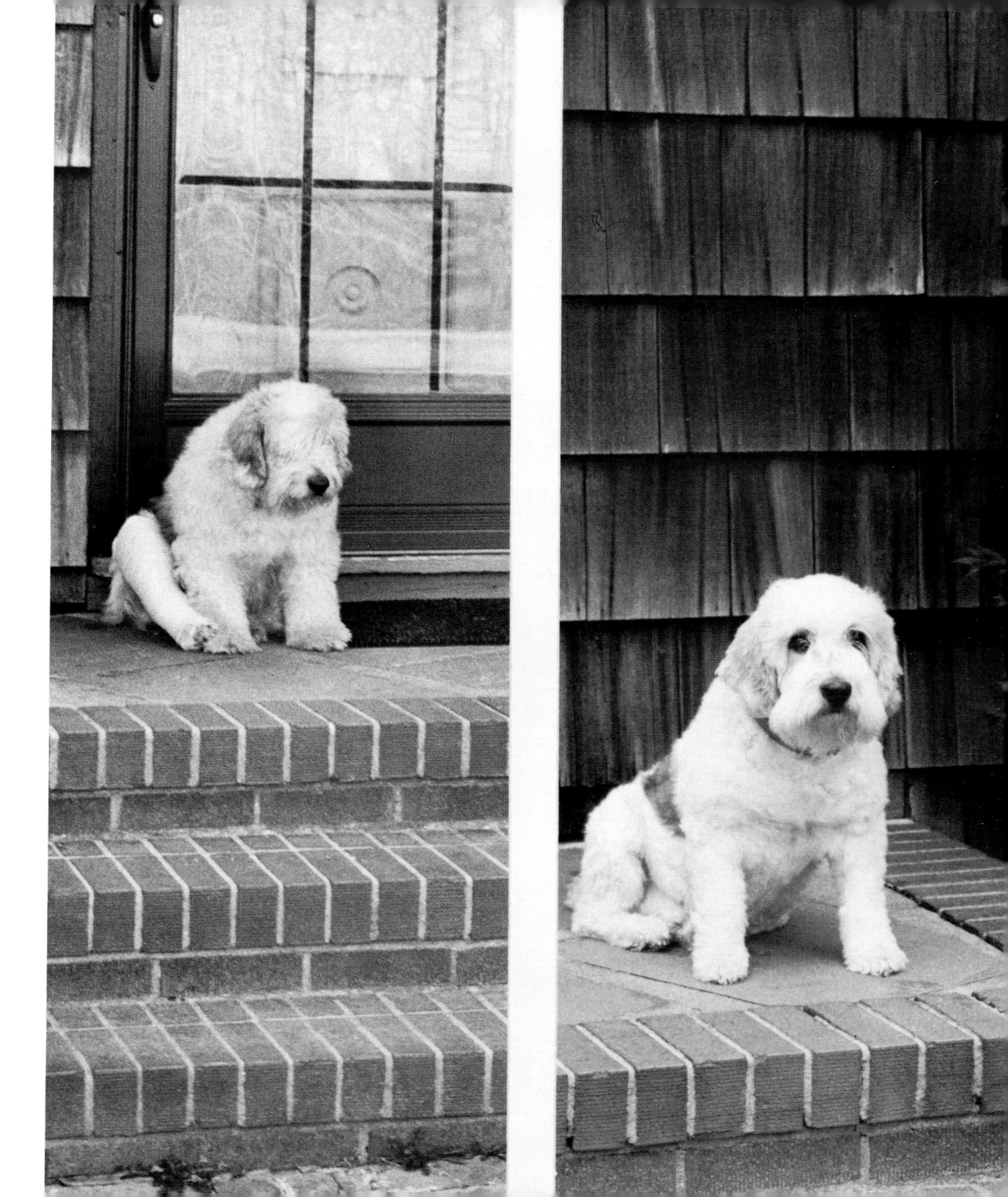

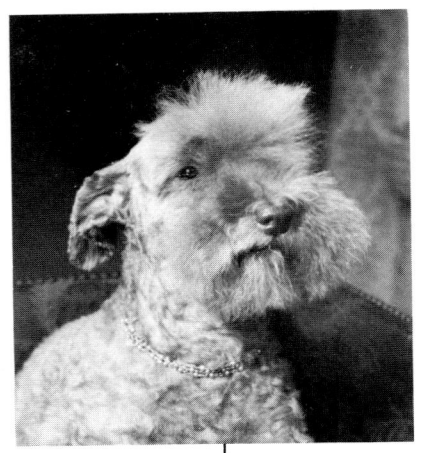

Poodle

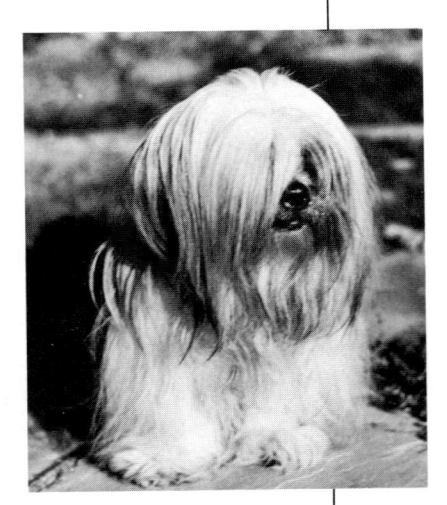

Lhasa Apso

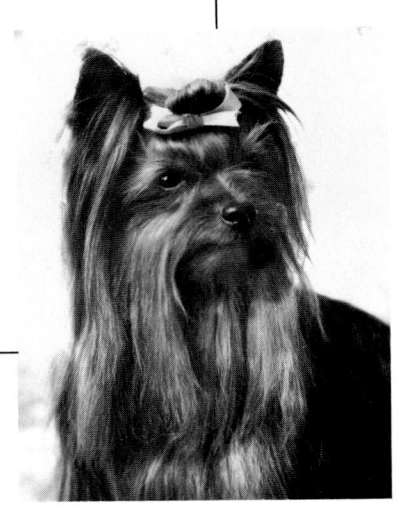

Yorkshire Terrier

Chipper was never told who his mother and father are, but he always suspected that he is "somebody." The lineup of his ancestors is very impressive.

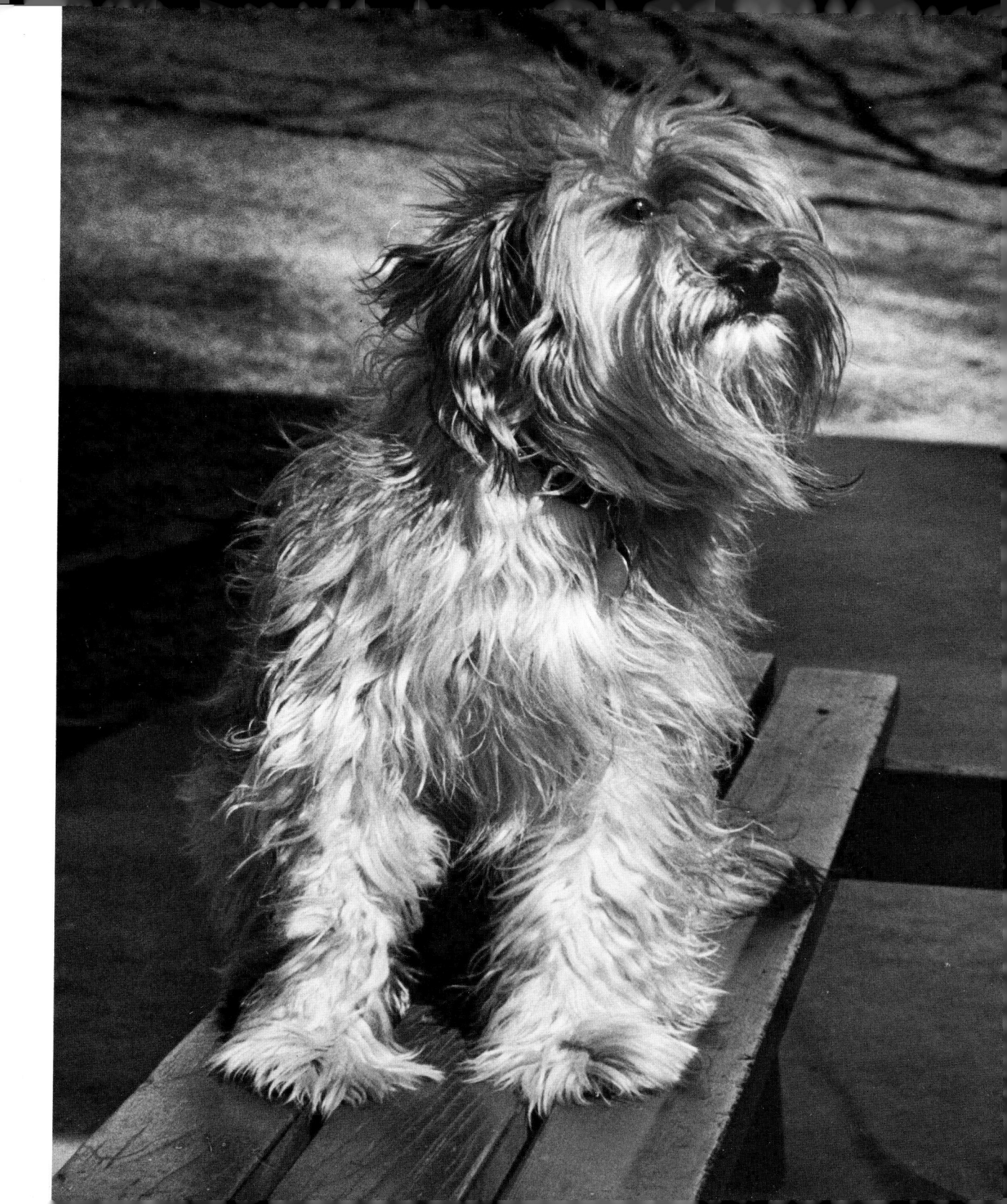

Bonnie likes to run on the beach, along the edge of the ocean. Sometimes she races through the waves. Bonnie inherited her love for the water from her father, a Yellow Labrador Retriever, and her grace and speed from her mother, an Irish Setter.

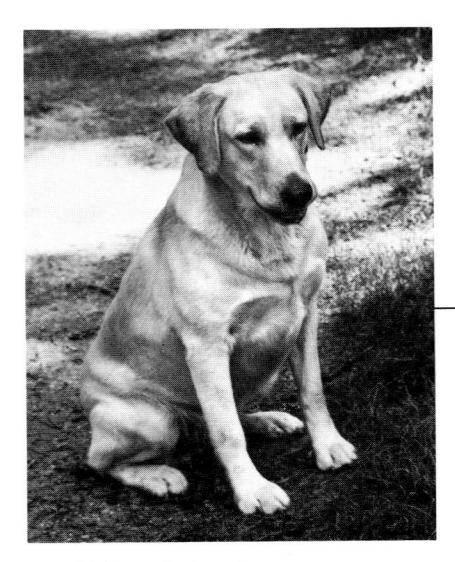

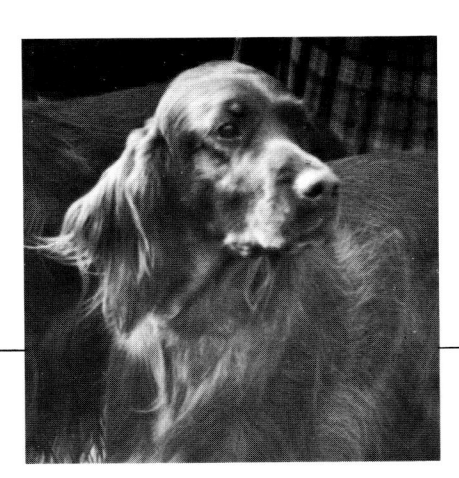

Irish Setter

Yellow Labrador

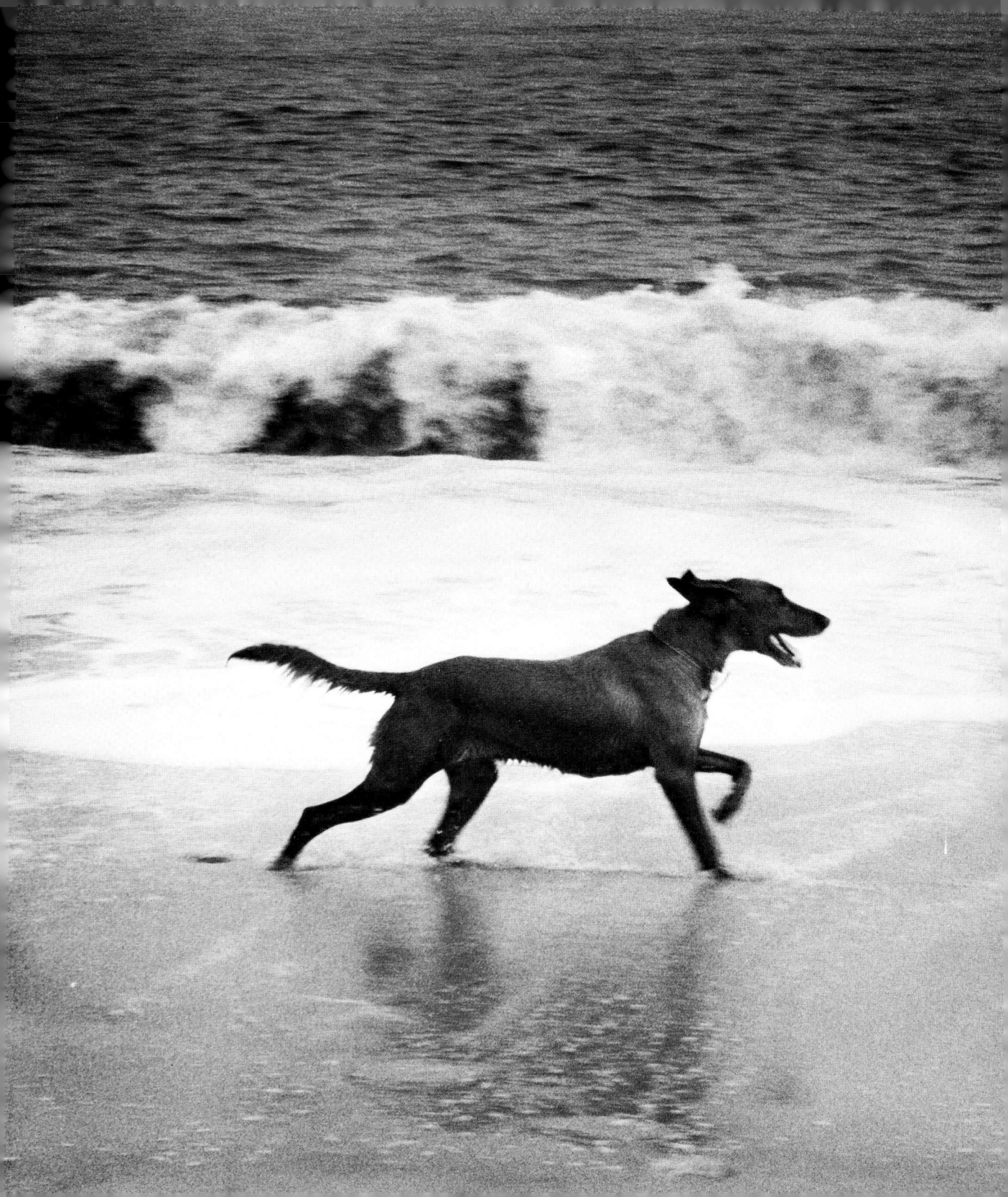

DeeDee is a good watchdog and a lovable pet. Her parents were German Shepherd and Collie. Everybody likes her except the neighbors' cats. Her sport is to chase them. Three cats live across the road and DeeDee's dream is someday to catch them. It will probably never happen because the cats scatter in three directions and vanish. Frustrated, DeeDee comes home to share the couch with Princess, the family cat.

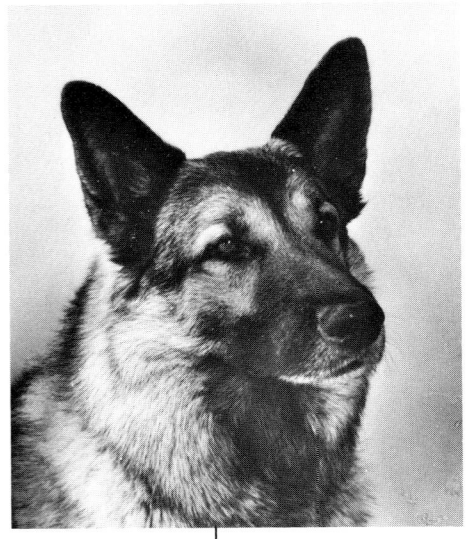

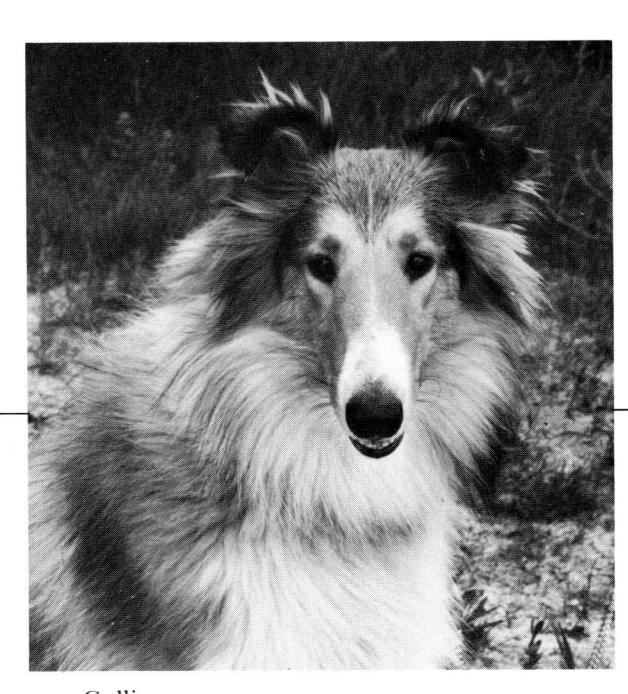

German Shepherd Dog

Collie

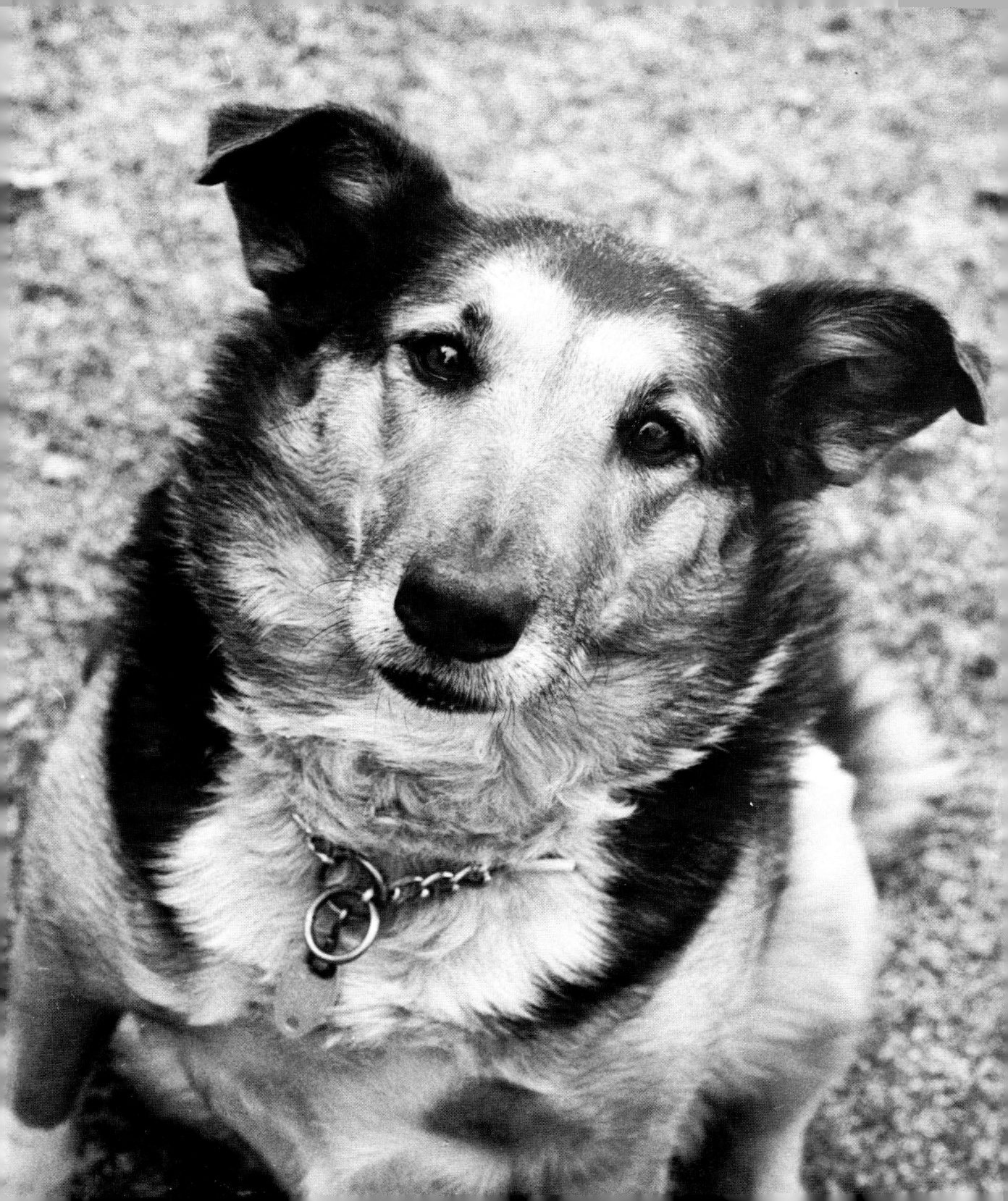

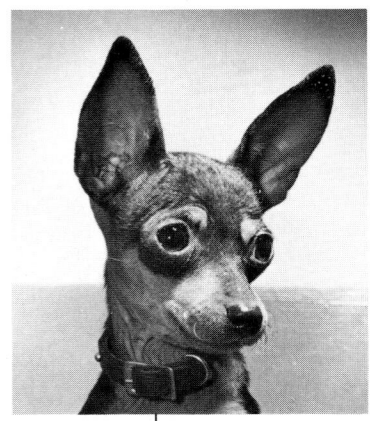

Toy Terrier

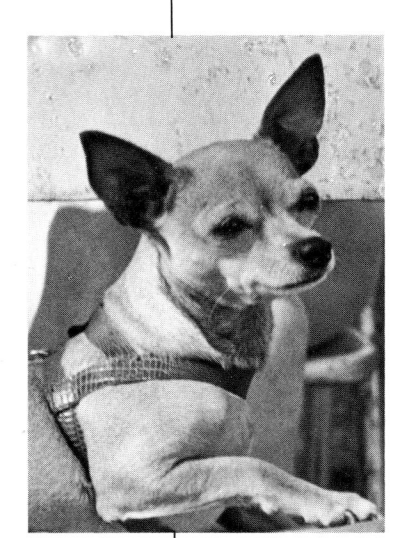

Buffy is not an average dog. He looks like an oversized Chihuahua. His movements and body have a strong resemblance to the Toy Terrier or a small Pinscher. Longer fur and a tail curled over his back indicate a long-haired ancestor with a curled tail, maybe a Keeshound. Socially Buffy is a hit—he sings in a melancholy way to the strings of the guitar.

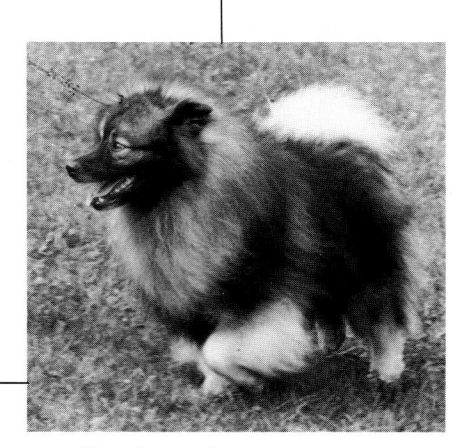

Chihuahua

Keeshound

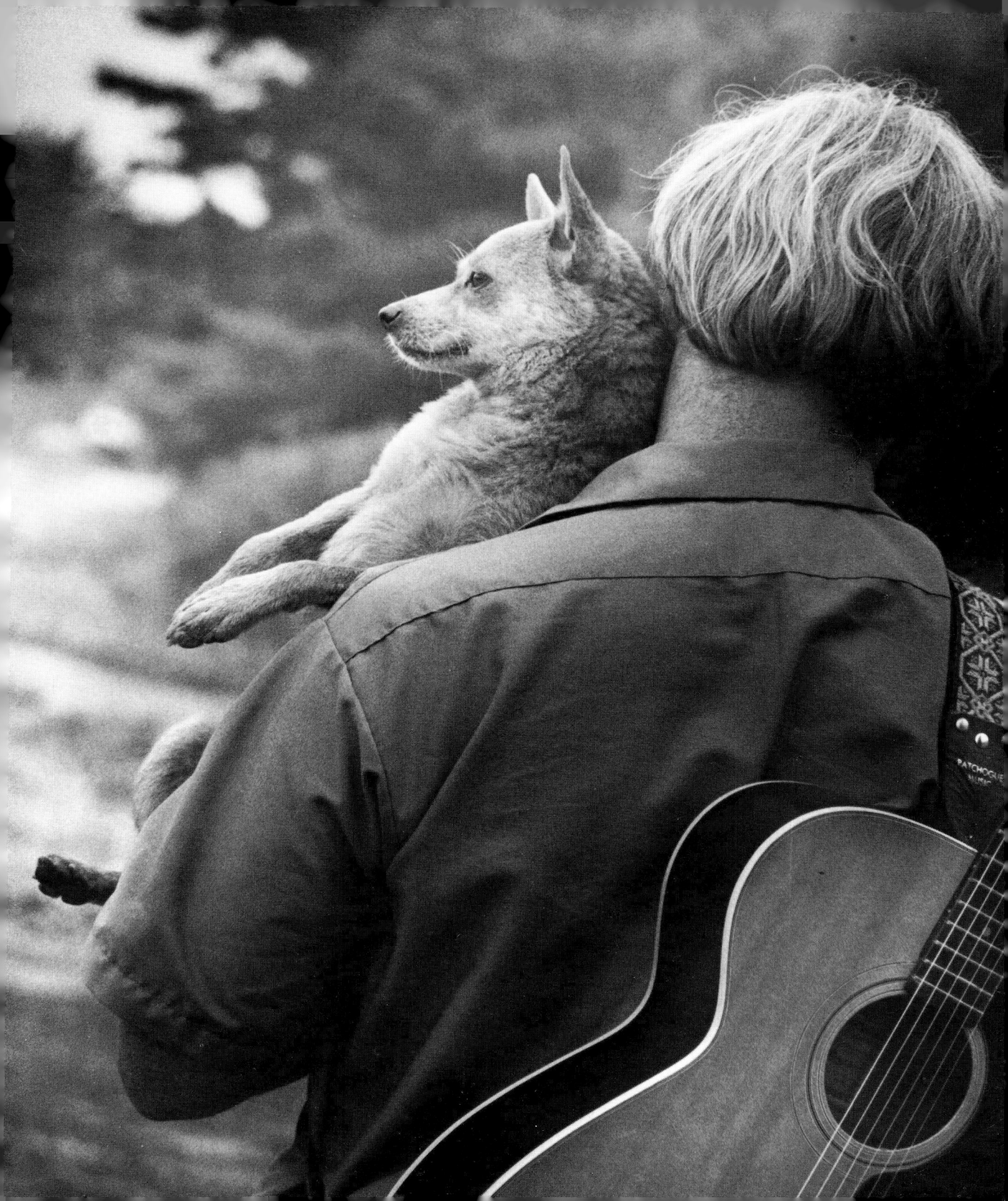

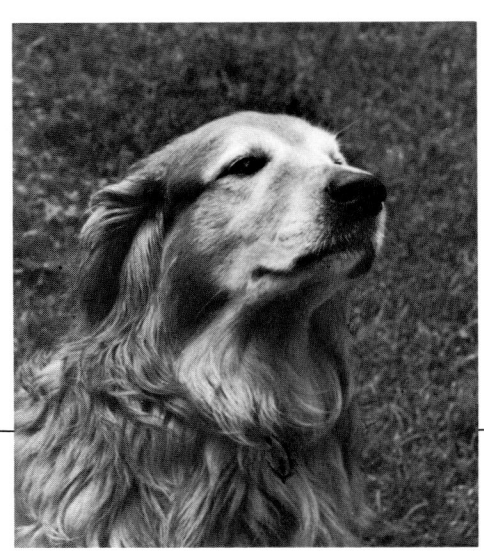

Golden Retriever

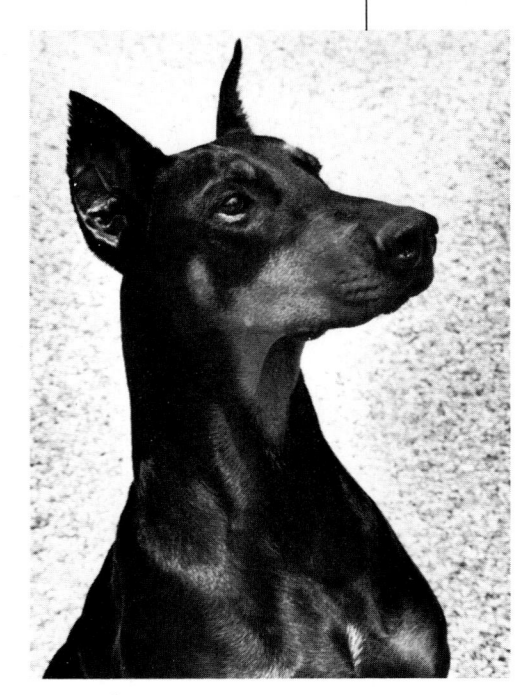

Doberman

Bunky lives in a big house,
but he also has his own small
white house, with a shingled
roof and his name over the entrance.
He is apparently a descendent of a
Doberman and a Golden Retriever.
When he is not busy playing with
a stick, he relaxes with a proud
look of a landowner aware of his
noble lineage.

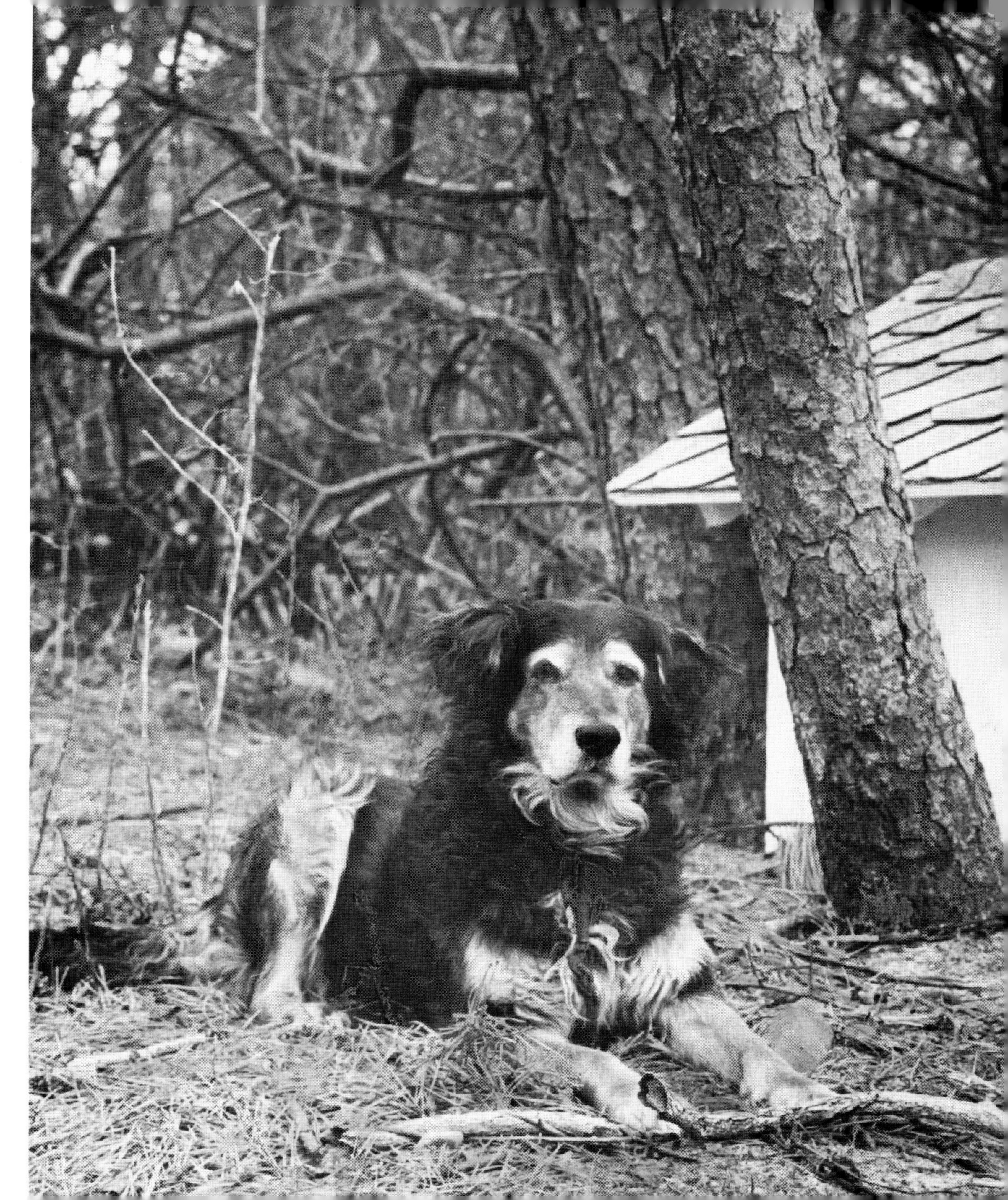

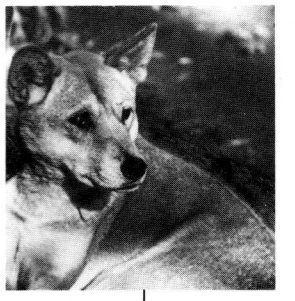

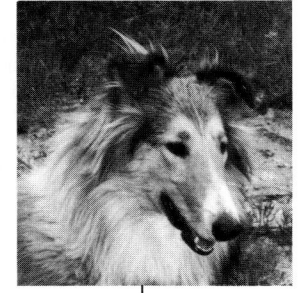

Dingo

Collie

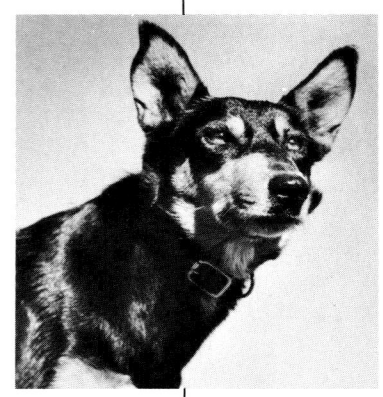

Australian Kelpie

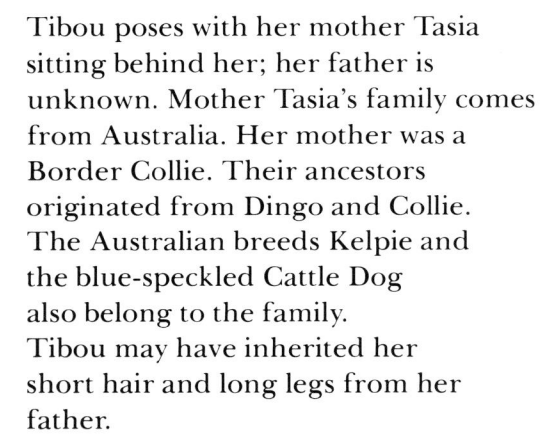

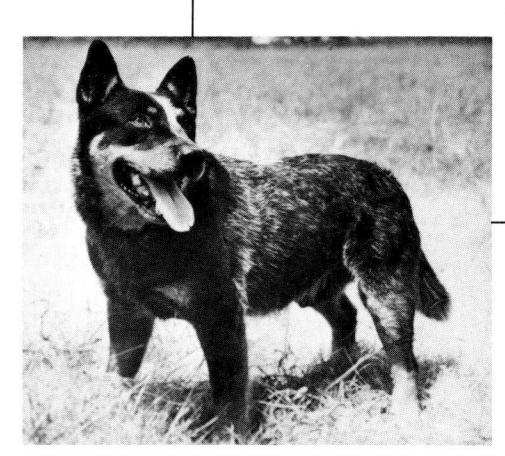

Australian Cattle Dog

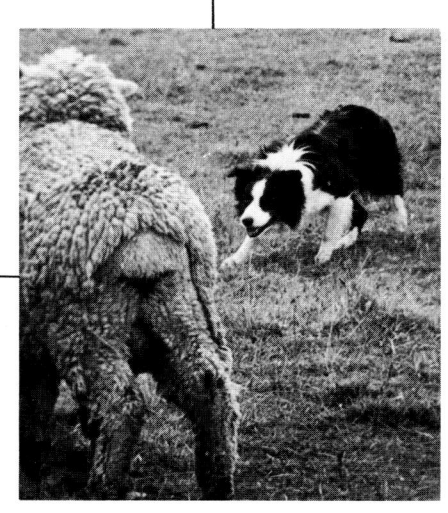

Border Collie

Tibou poses with her mother Tasia sitting behind her; her father is unknown. Mother Tasia's family comes from Australia. Her mother was a Border Collie. Their ancestors originated from Dingo and Collie. The Australian breeds Kelpie and the blue-speckled Cattle Dog also belong to the family. Tibou may have inherited her short hair and long legs from her father.

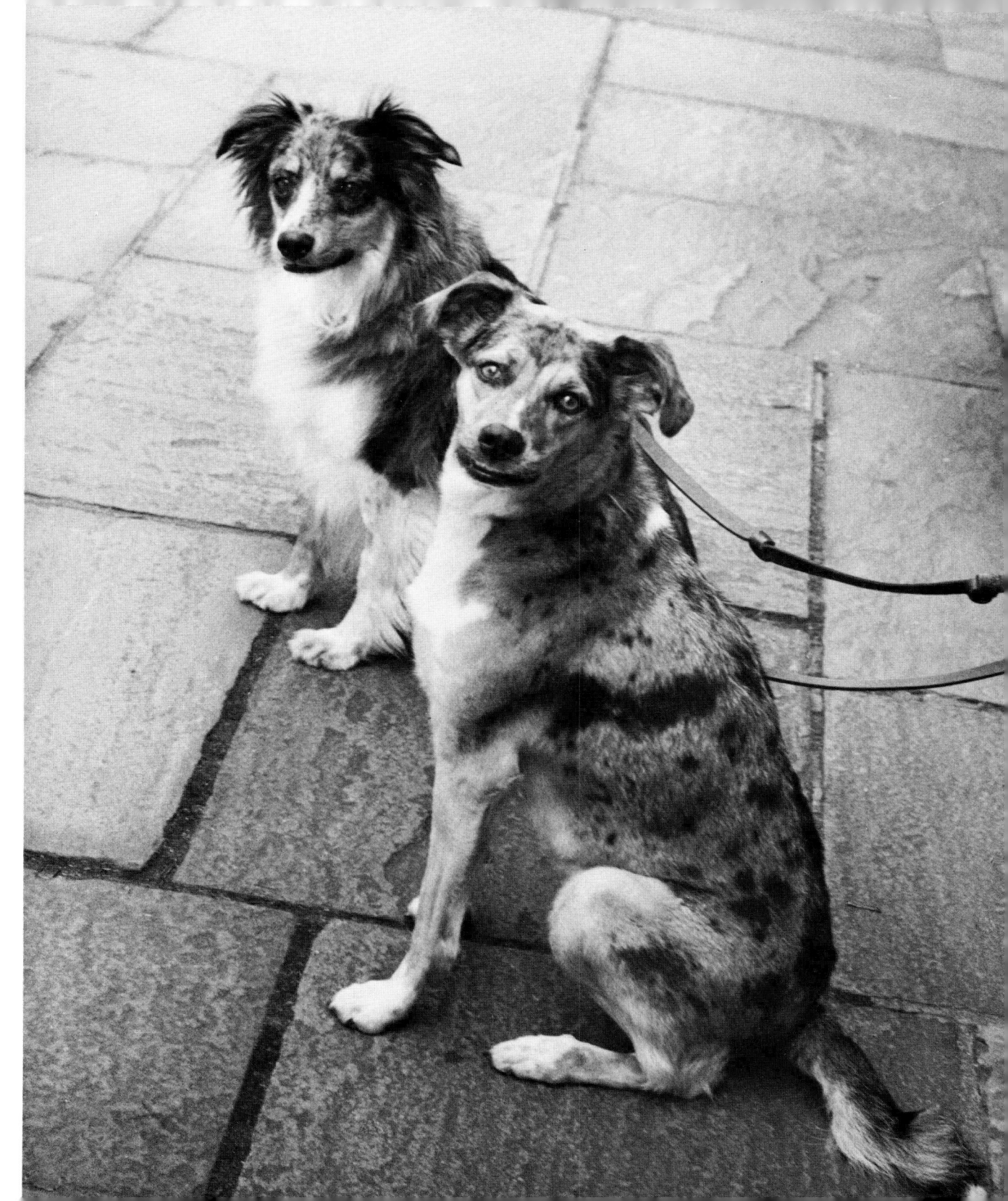

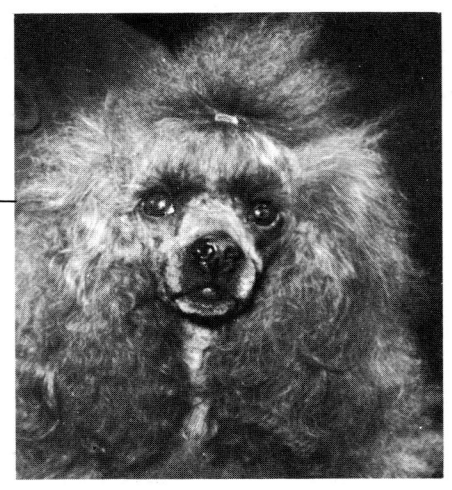

Poodle

Tootsie is grown up but she
looks and acts like a puppy.
Her parents were a Poodle and a Chow.
She likes to play and eat.
The sound of popping popcorn
makes her come running to the
kitchen. She is addicted to
cookies and, in anticipation
of getting some, can
stand up indefinitely.
If the wait is too long, she
topples over, but next moment
is up again—and then usually
gets a cookie.

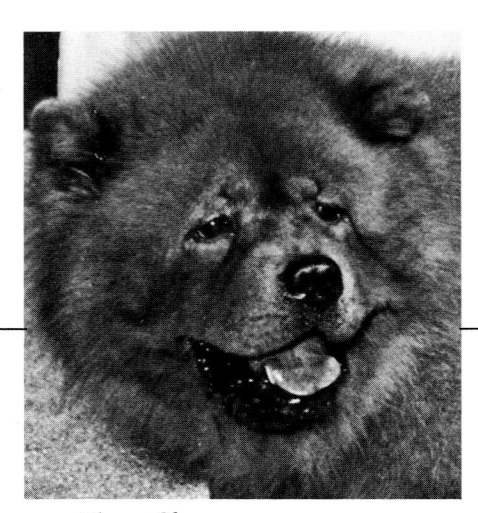

Chow Chow

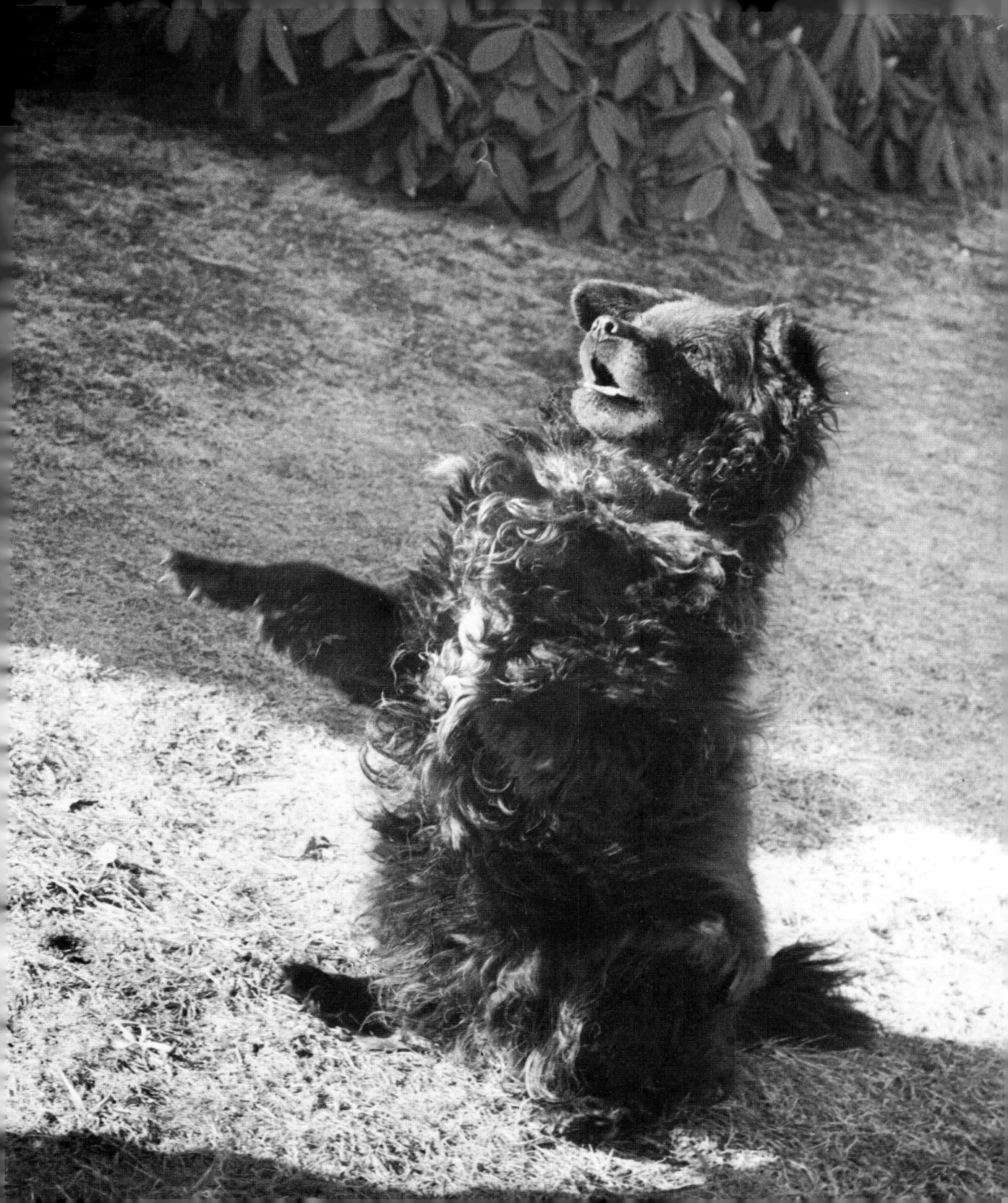

Moffet had an unusual childhood. His father was a Beagle. The mother, a Wirehaired Fox Terrier, refused to nurse Moffett. It so happened that the cat Harriet had a litter and was nursing her kittens—Moffet was added to her family. Harriet adopted the new "kitten" and Moffet found a mother. Now, when the "kitten" is grown-up, big and strong, Harriet avoids his rugged games. Sometimes she goes up a tree.

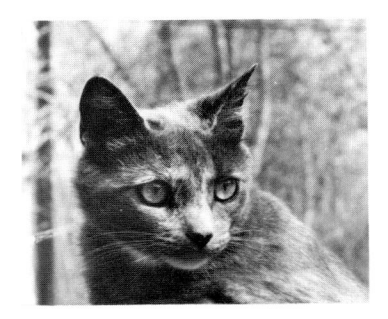

Harriet, foster mother

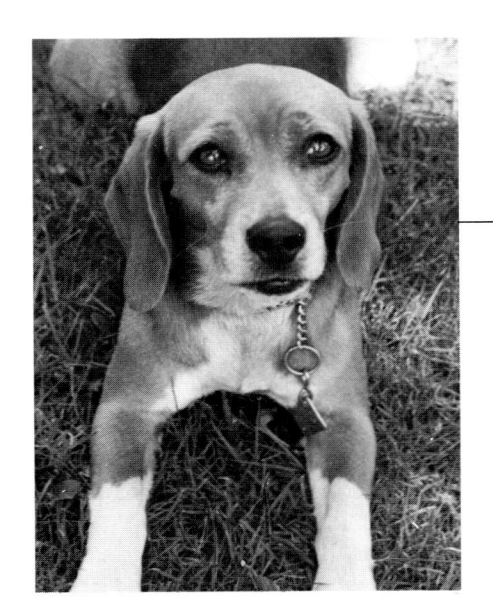

Beagle

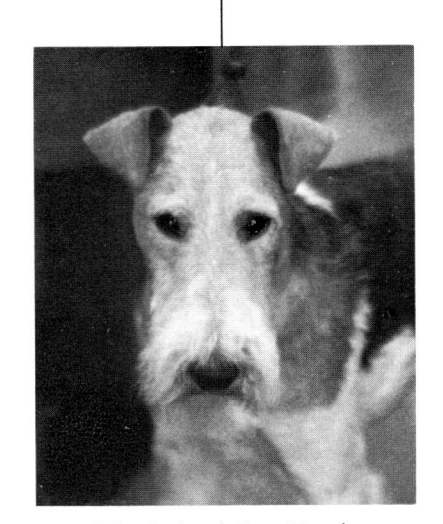

Wirehaired Fox Terrier

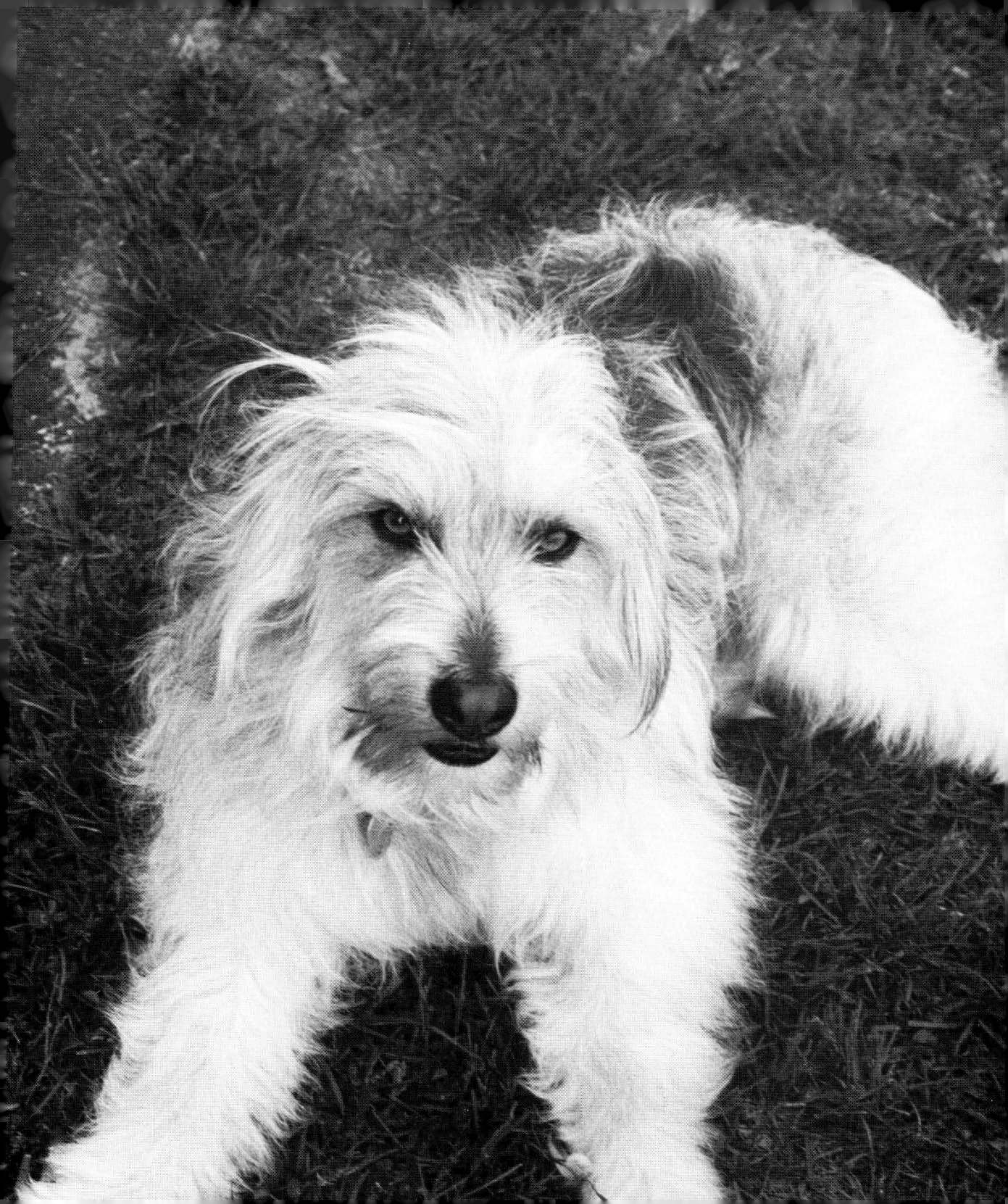

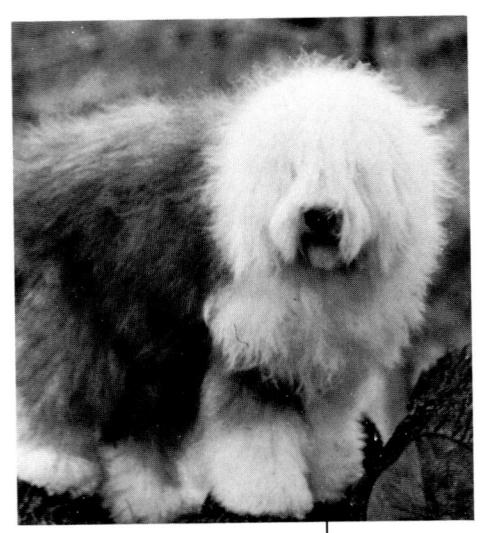

Brutus is good-natured,
big and woolly.
Nobody is sure
who his parents are.
The Old English Sheepdog
and the Otter Hound
are two of his ancestors.
He does not hunt otters
or take care of sheep—
Brutus is a pet.

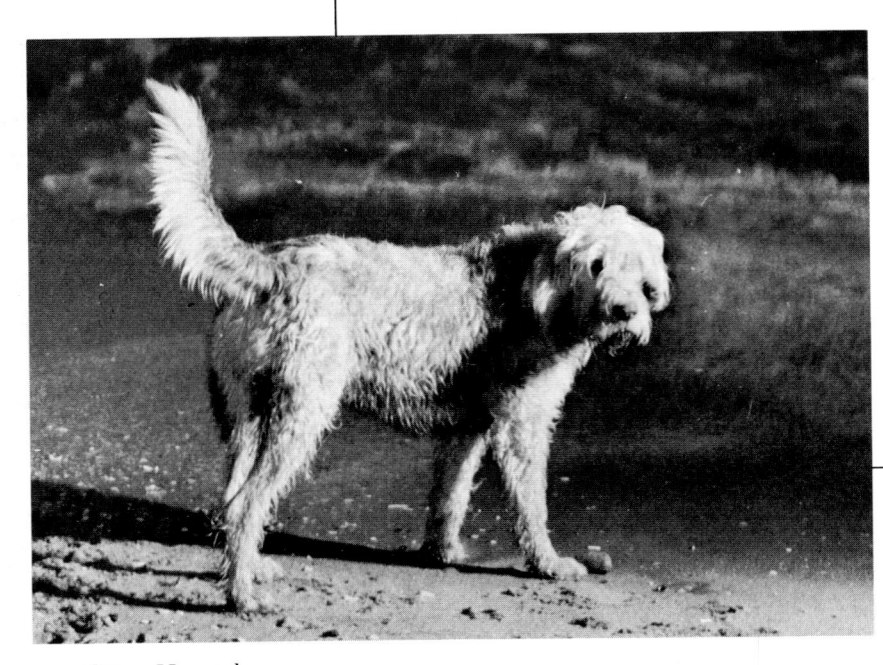

Old English Sheepdog

Otter Hound

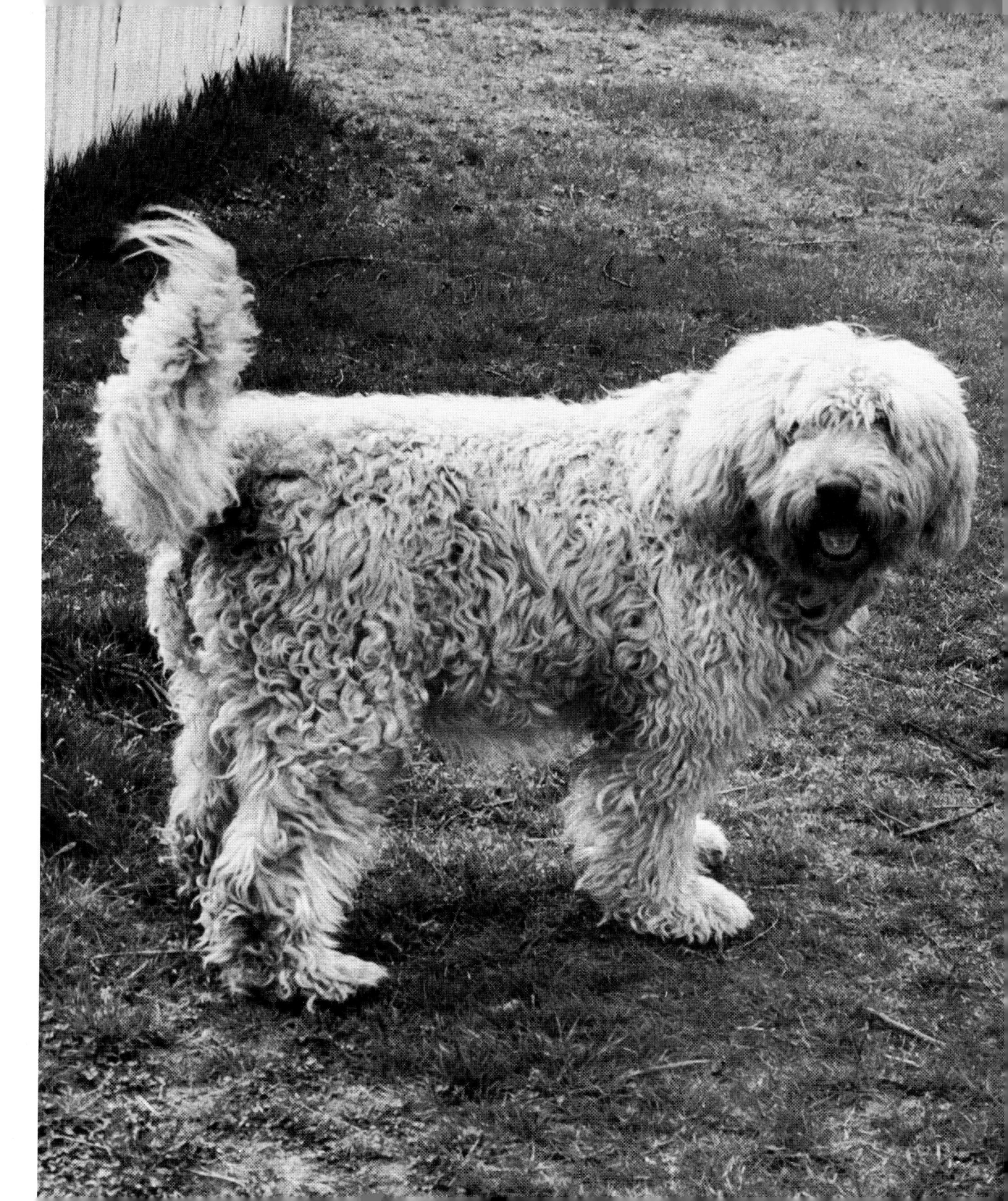

Misty leads a busy life.
Every morning she takes her place
at the family fruit-and-vegetable
road stand. She inspects the second
stand, miles away, occasionally.
Misty feels just as important
guarding her watermelons as her
ancestor the Puli does guarding
his sheep. From her other ancestor,
the Schnauzer, she inherited devotion
and whiskers.

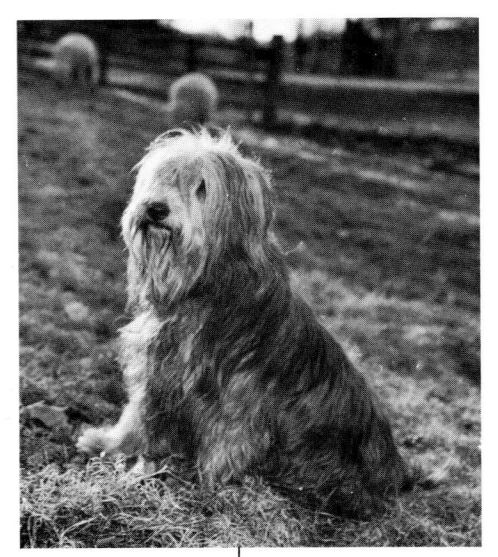

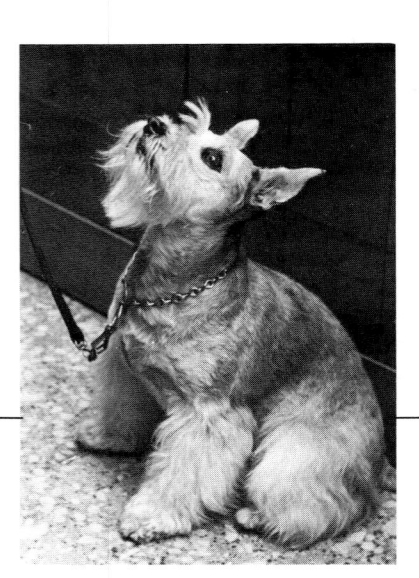

Puli

Schnauzer

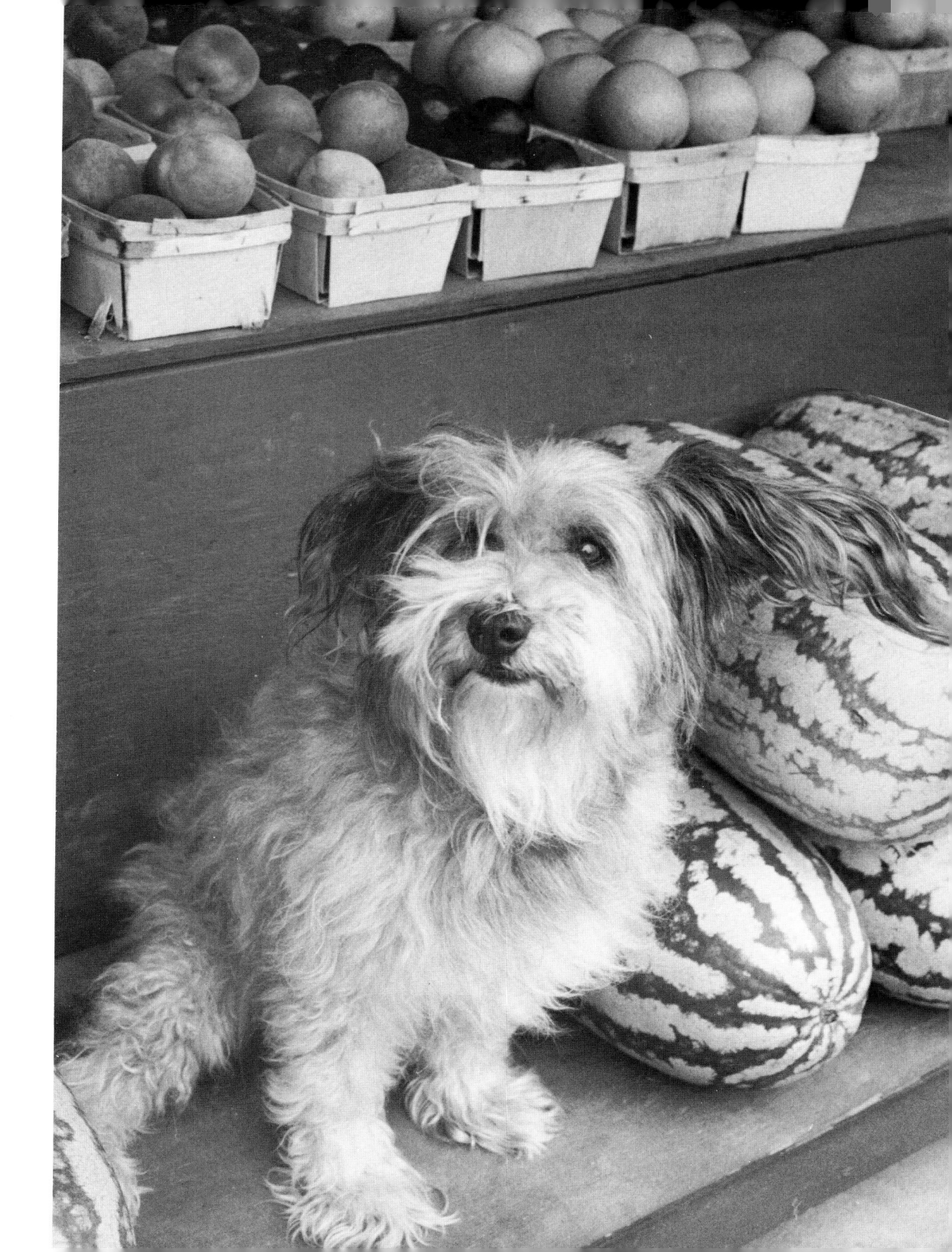

Furry and Foxy are sisters. Among their ancestors are the Whippet and the White Shepherd. They grew up together but their personalities are very different. Furry is an alert watchdog, ready to face and intimidate strangers. She also likes to bark. Foxy is timid, shy, and never barks. They live, sleep, and eat together. Never away from each other, they are as close as twins could be. When Furry has her nails trimmed, Foxy cries.

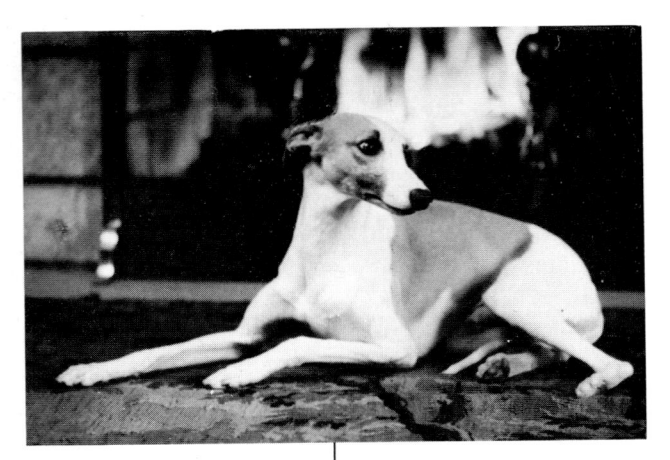

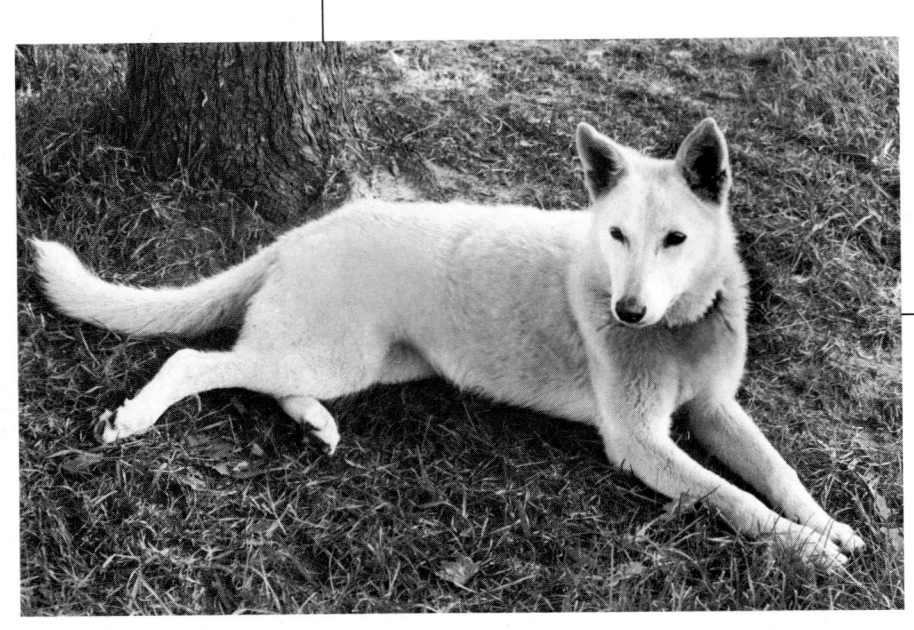

Whippet

White Shepherd

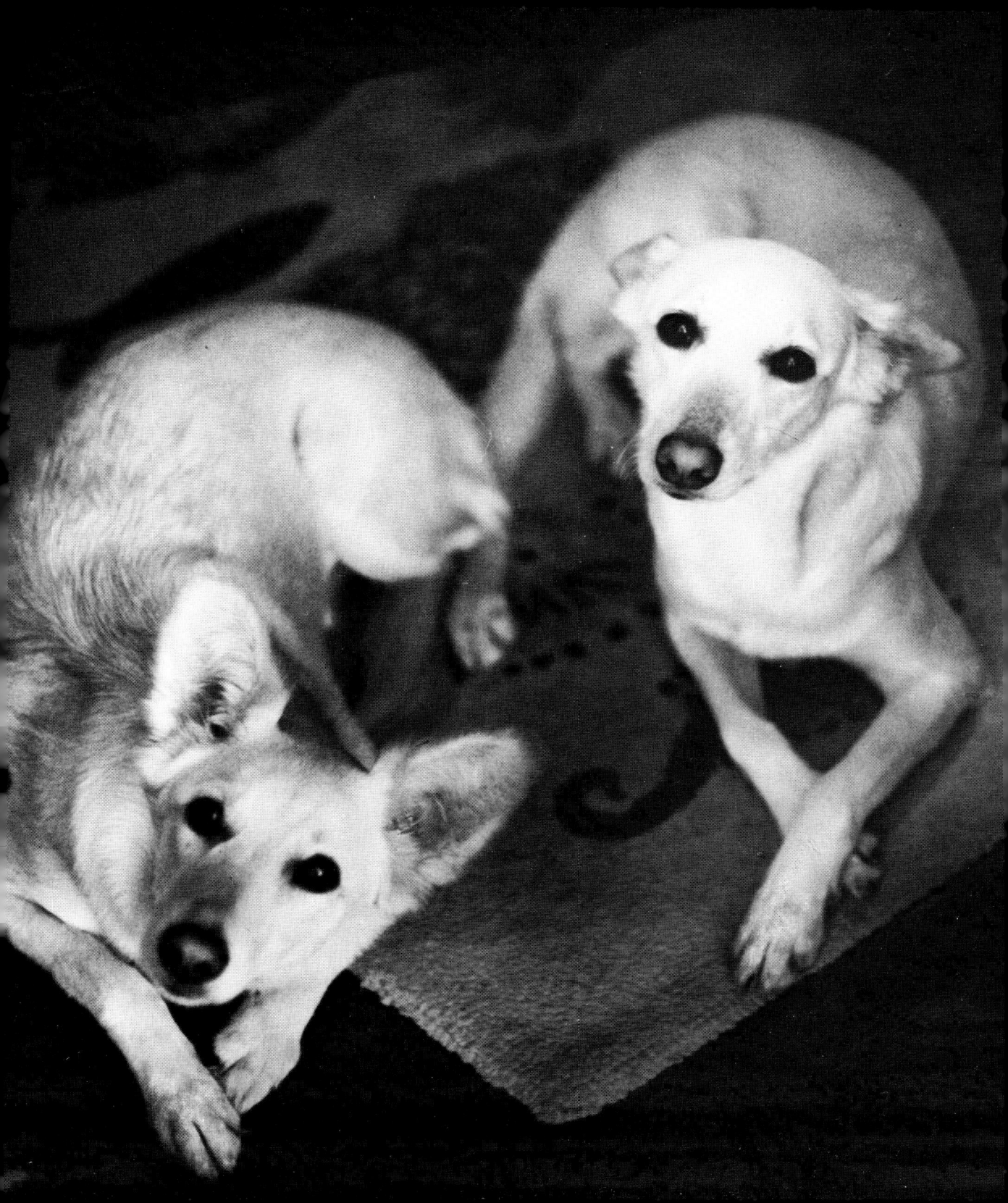

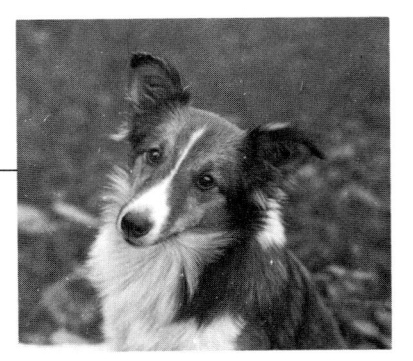

Missy has looks and personality—
nobody can ask for more.
Her mother was a Shetland Sheepdog, her
father was a Corgi or a Dachshund,
both breeds are in her ancestry.
She was born in the country, moved
later to the big town—now Missy
is a well-adjusted city dog,
nothing can surprise her.

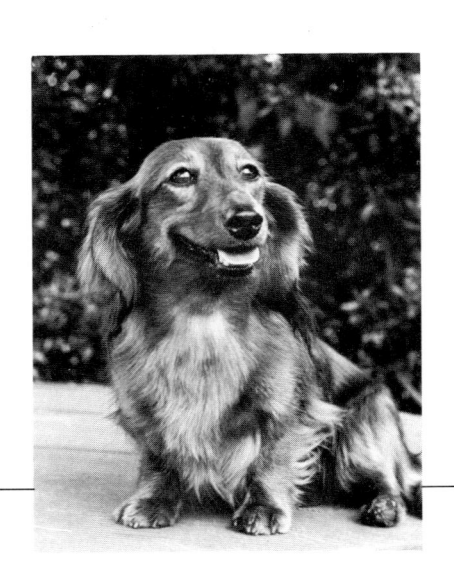

Shetland Sheepdog

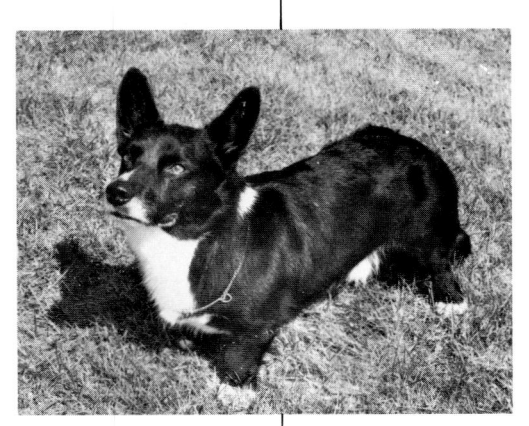

Welsh Corgi Cardigan

Miniature Long-haired
Dachshund

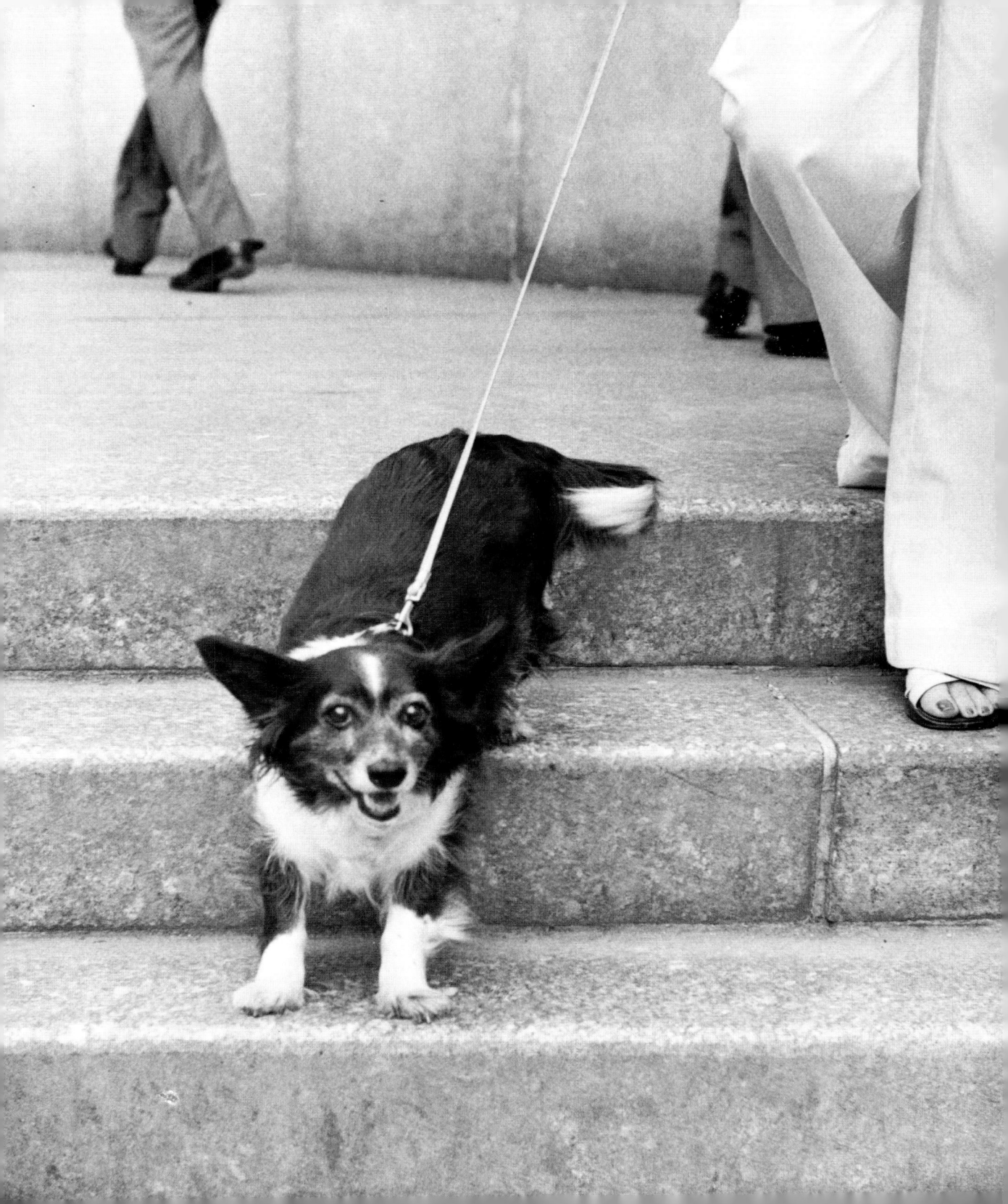

Jake is the son of a Dalmatian and a German Short-haired Pointer. He has never been on a fire engine racing to a fire or pointed at game on hunting trips.
He is a pet and satisfied with nothing more exciting than a ride in the car to the neighborhood shopping center. He is the only dog in the family and that's the way he likes it.

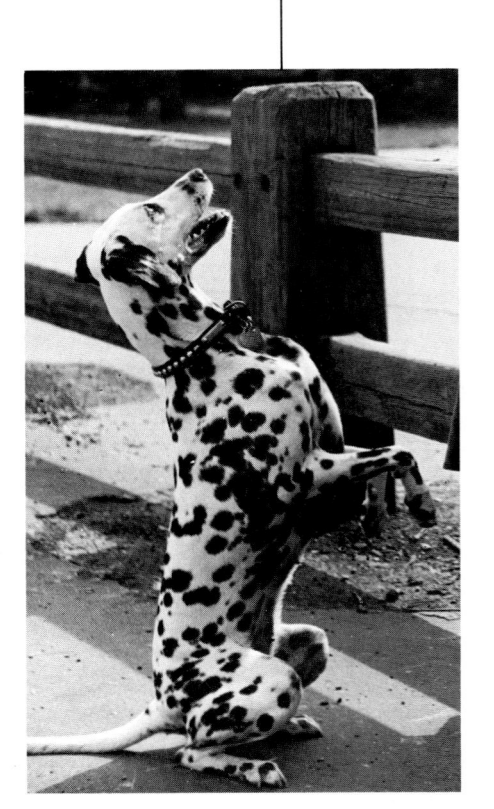

German Short-haired Pointer

Dalmatian

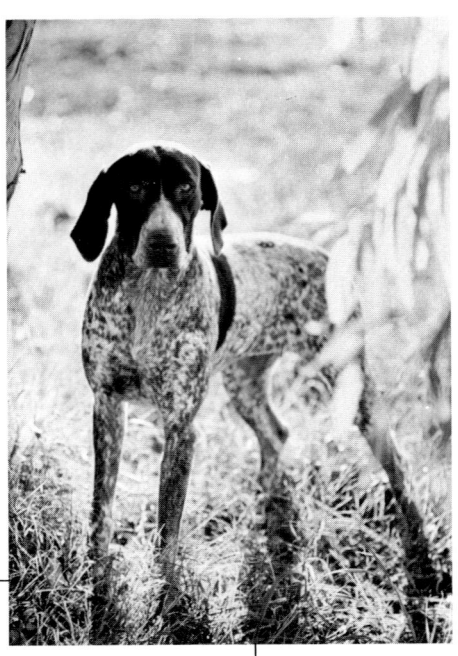

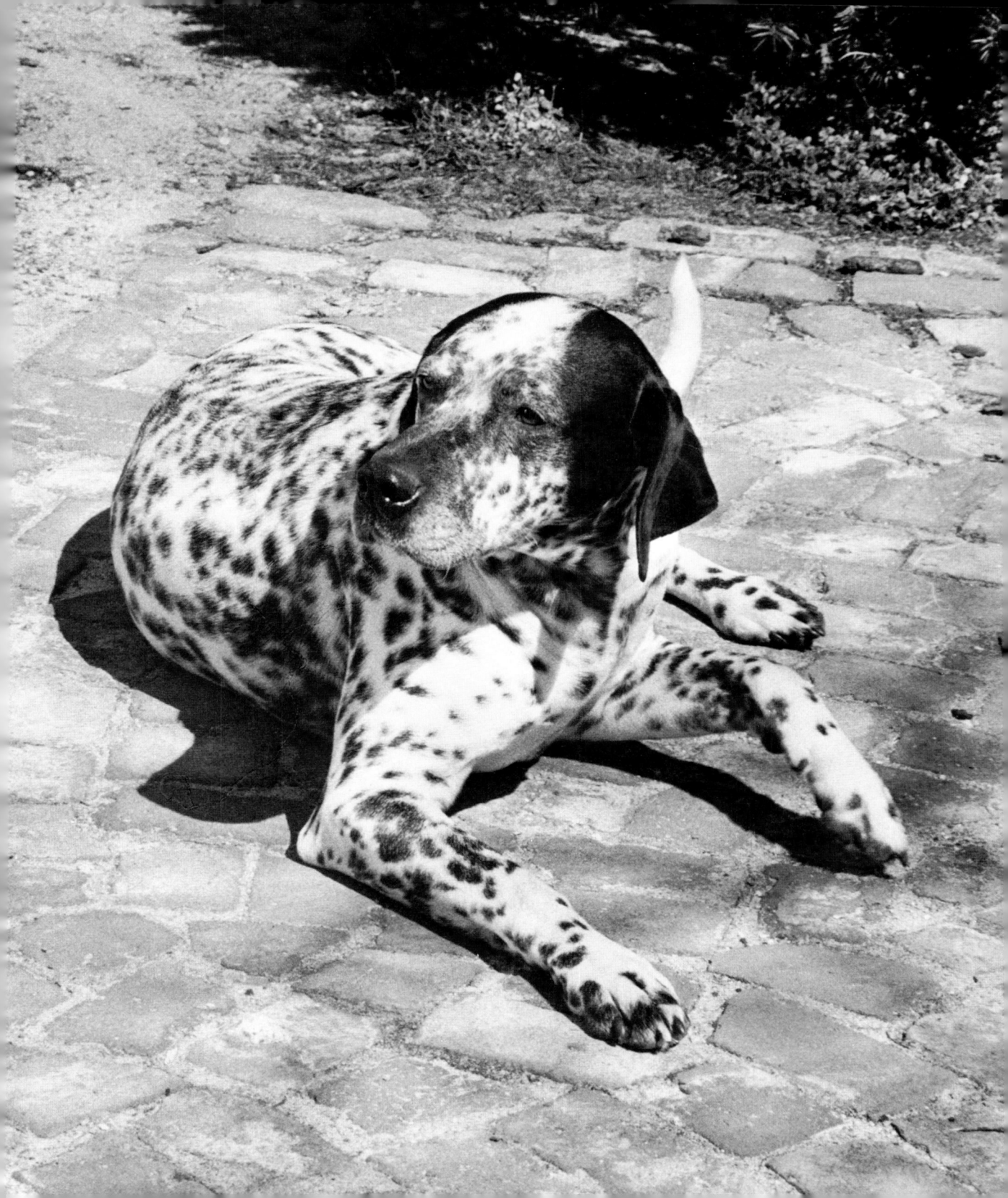

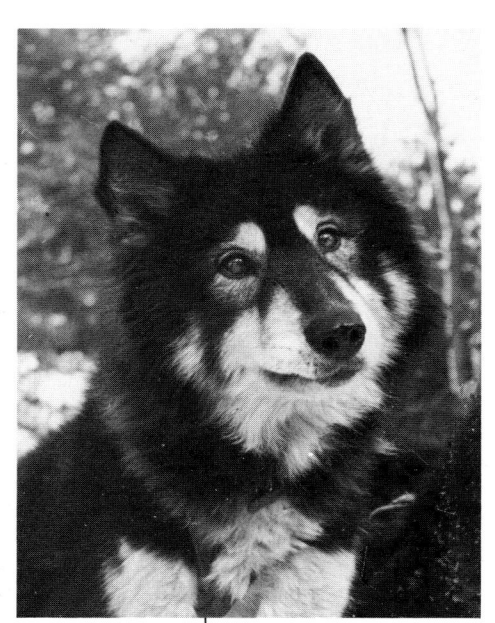

Jenny came from Alaska, her mother was a Collie, her father a Canadian Husky. She is shy and suspicious of strangers. She has lived through bad times and her eyes tell about it.

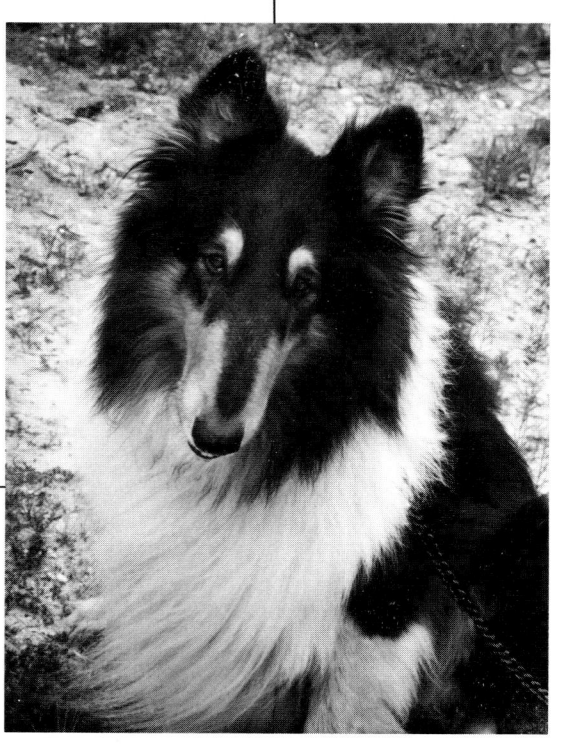

Canadian Husky

Collie

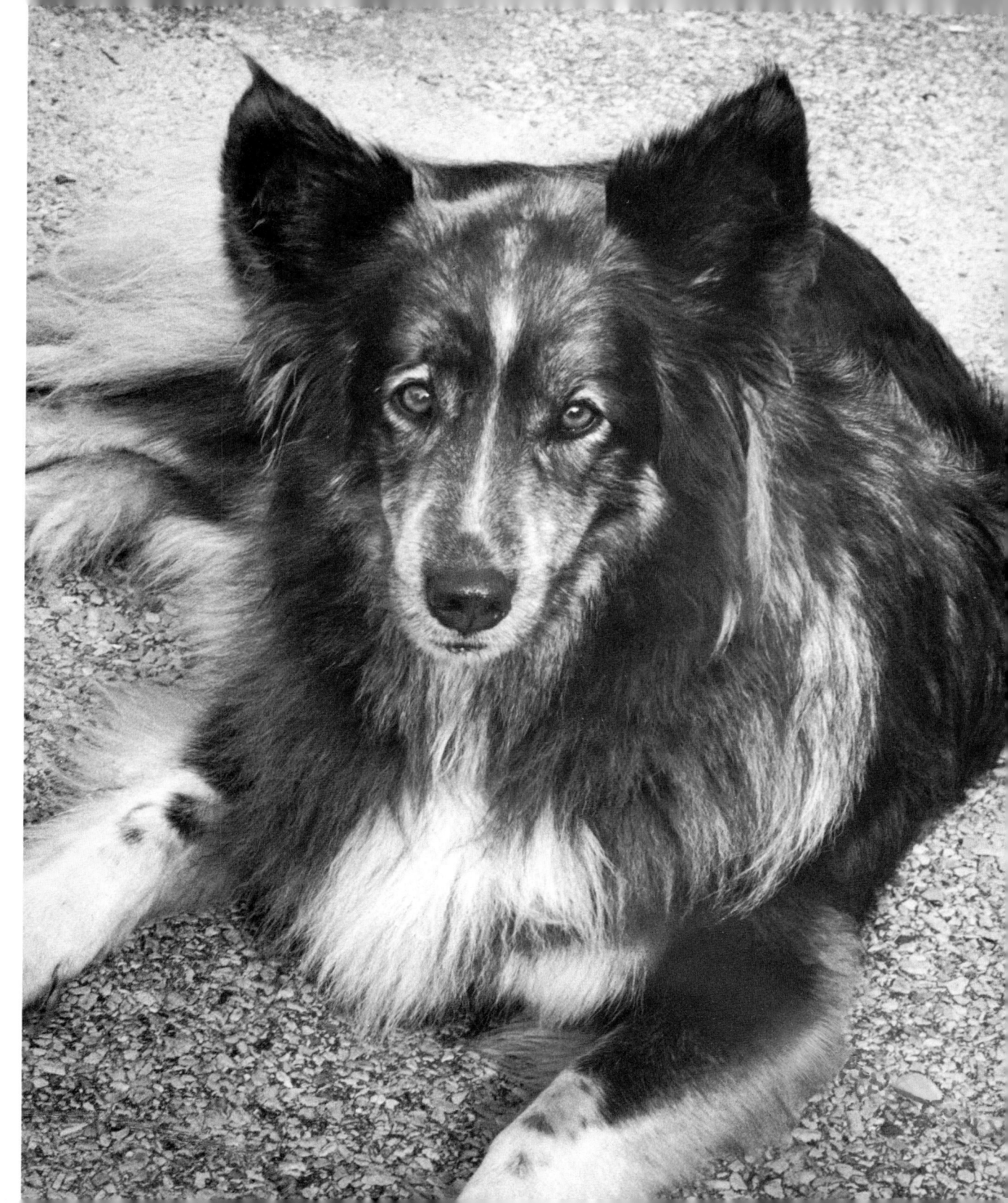

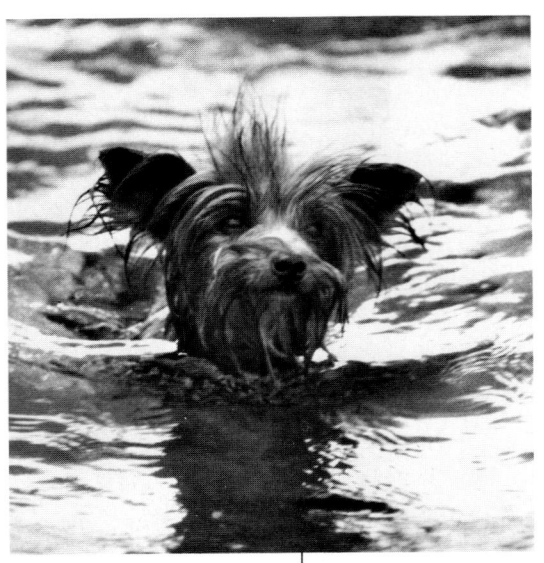

Tex is a Texan.
His parents were
a Long-haired Dachshund
and a Yorkshire Terrier.
He has an engaging personality,
and makes friends easily. While
he lives close to the sea,
he hates swimming. Once,
during a storm, when the
family boat was sinking,
Tex was saved first.

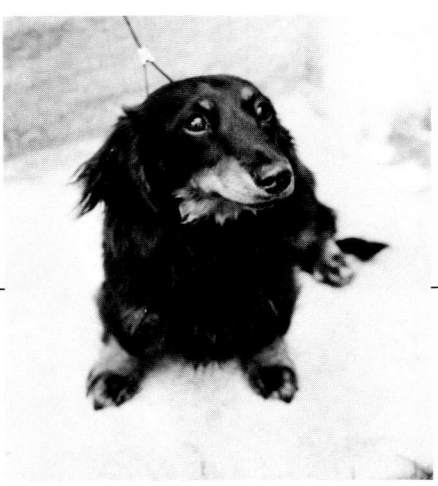

Yorkshire Terrier

Long-haired Dachshund

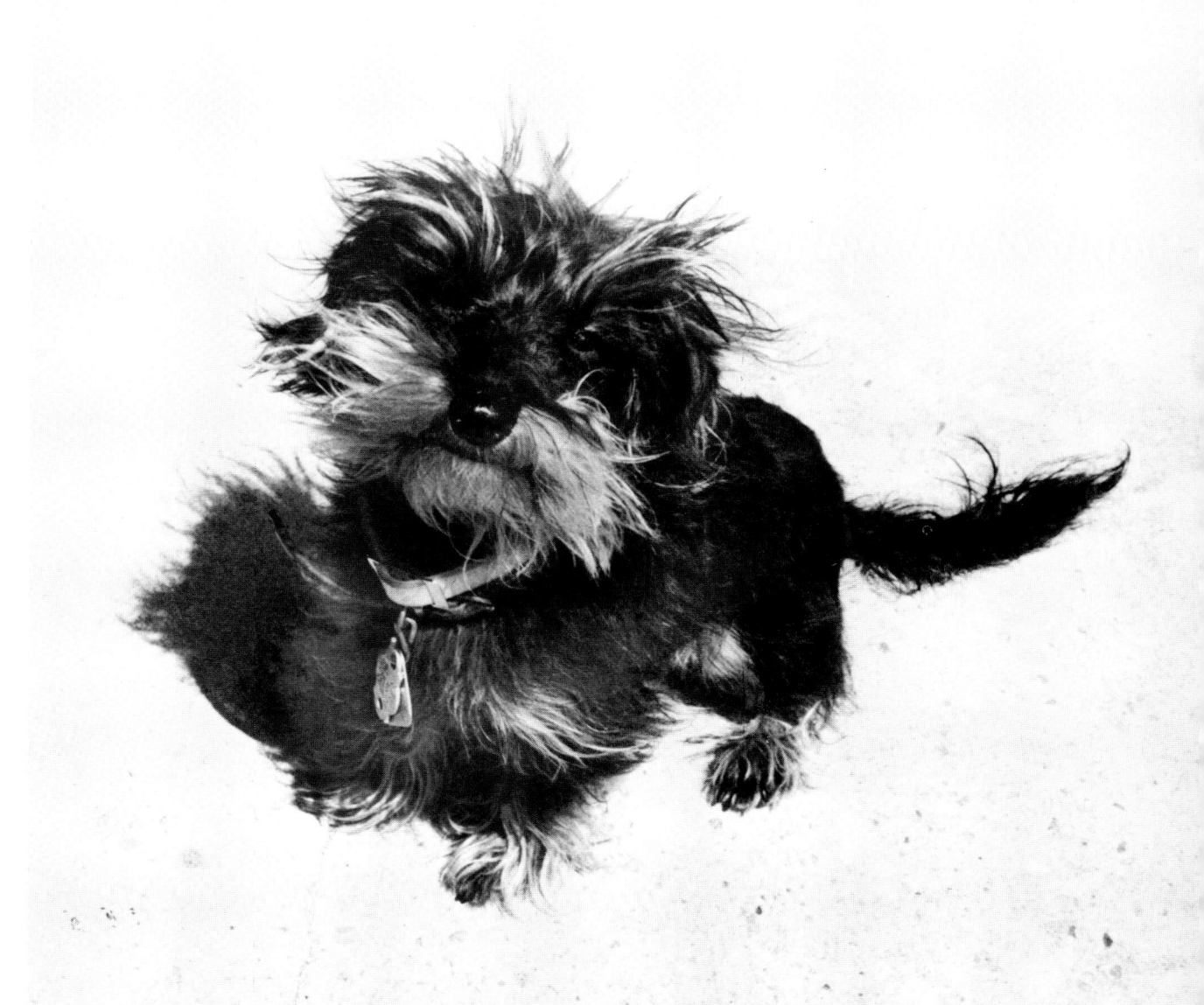

Meagan was born to a Great Dane
and a St. Bernard.
Her body is mostly Great Dane,
her head and disposition remind one
of a St. Bernard. Meagan is young
and inexperienced. She does not
know her size and strength.
She likes to play with a little
Yorkshire Terrier, Penelope,
but the pleasure is not mutual.

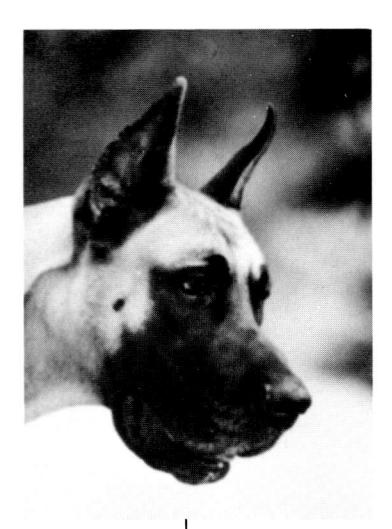

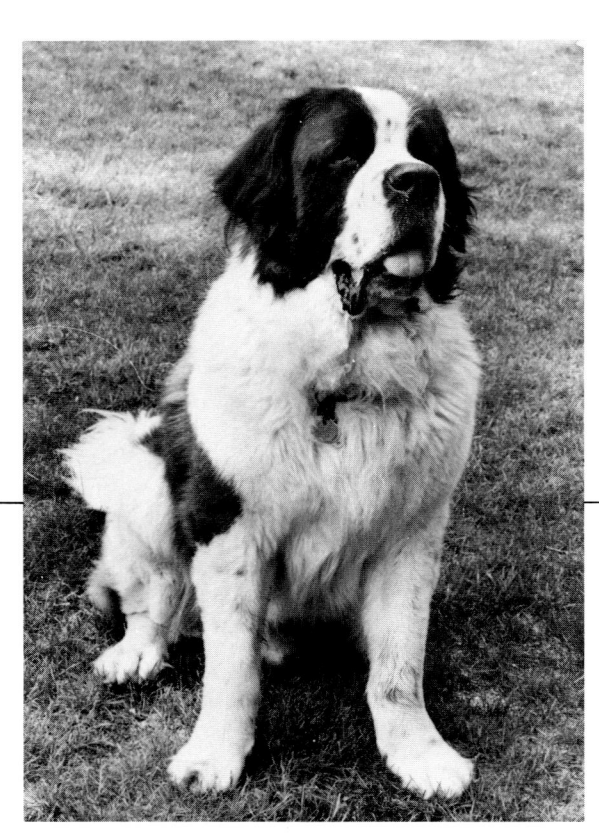

Great Dane

St. Bernard

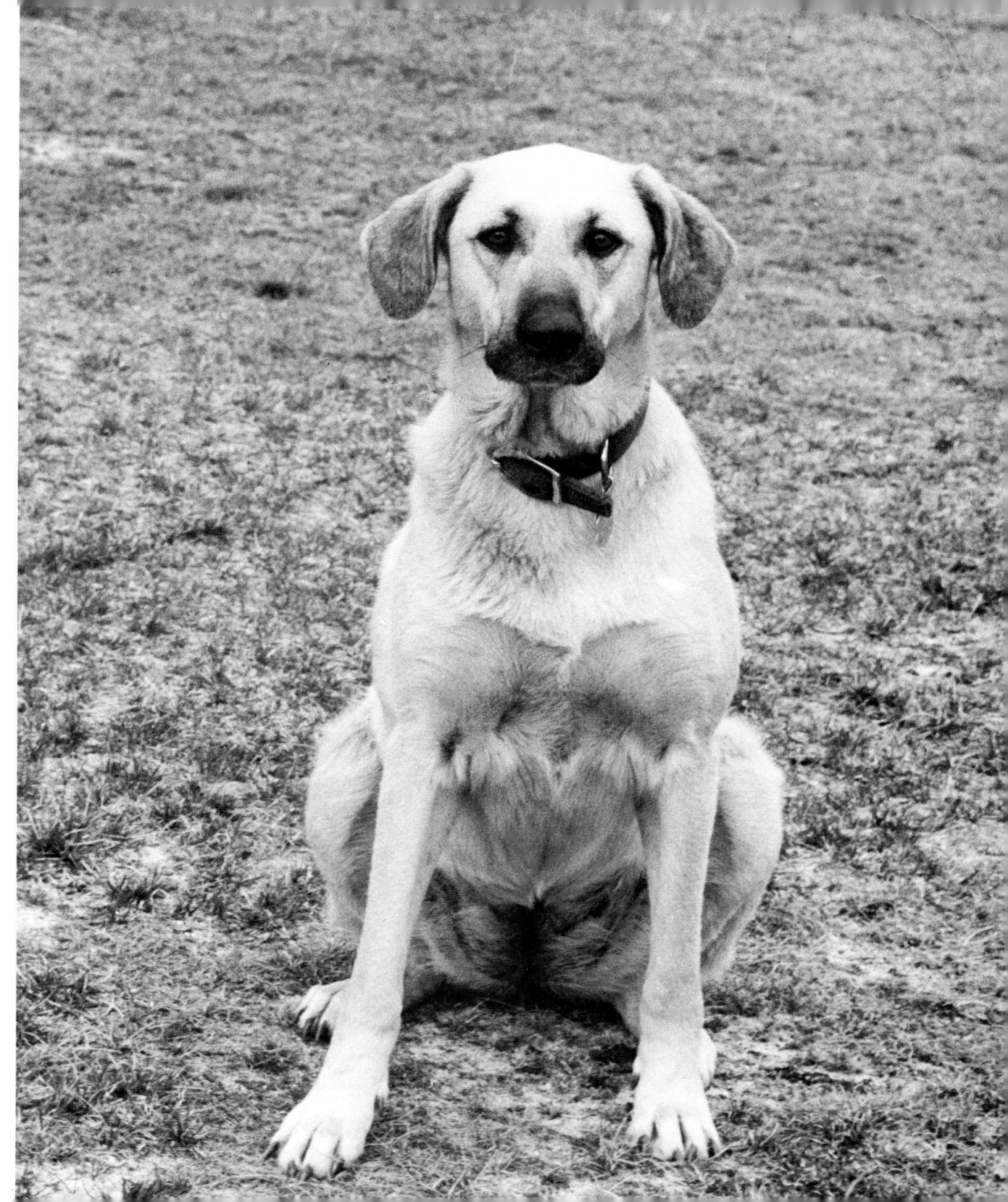

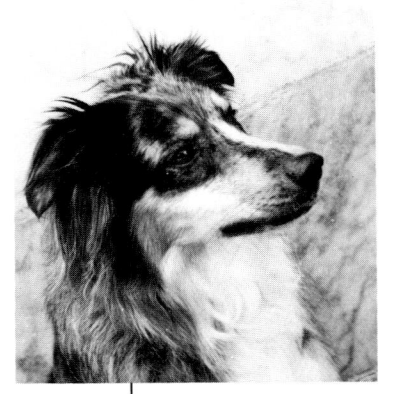

Australian Sheepdog

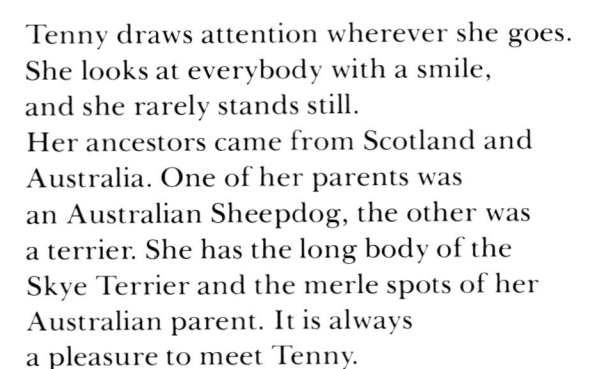

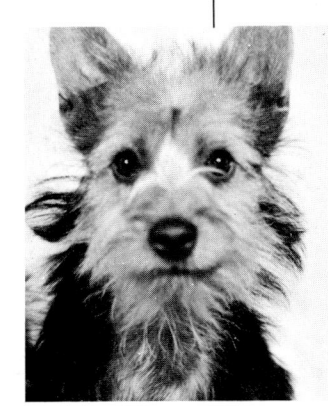

Tenny draws attention wherever she goes.
She looks at everybody with a smile,
and she rarely stands still.
Her ancestors came from Scotland and
Australia. One of her parents was
an Australian Sheepdog, the other was
a terrier. She has the long body of the
Skye Terrier and the merle spots of her
Australian parent. It is always
a pleasure to meet Tenny.

Australian Terrier

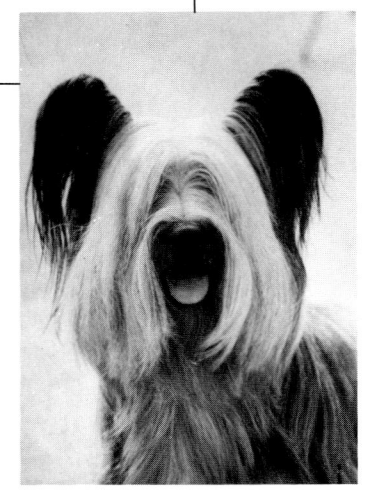

Skye Terrier

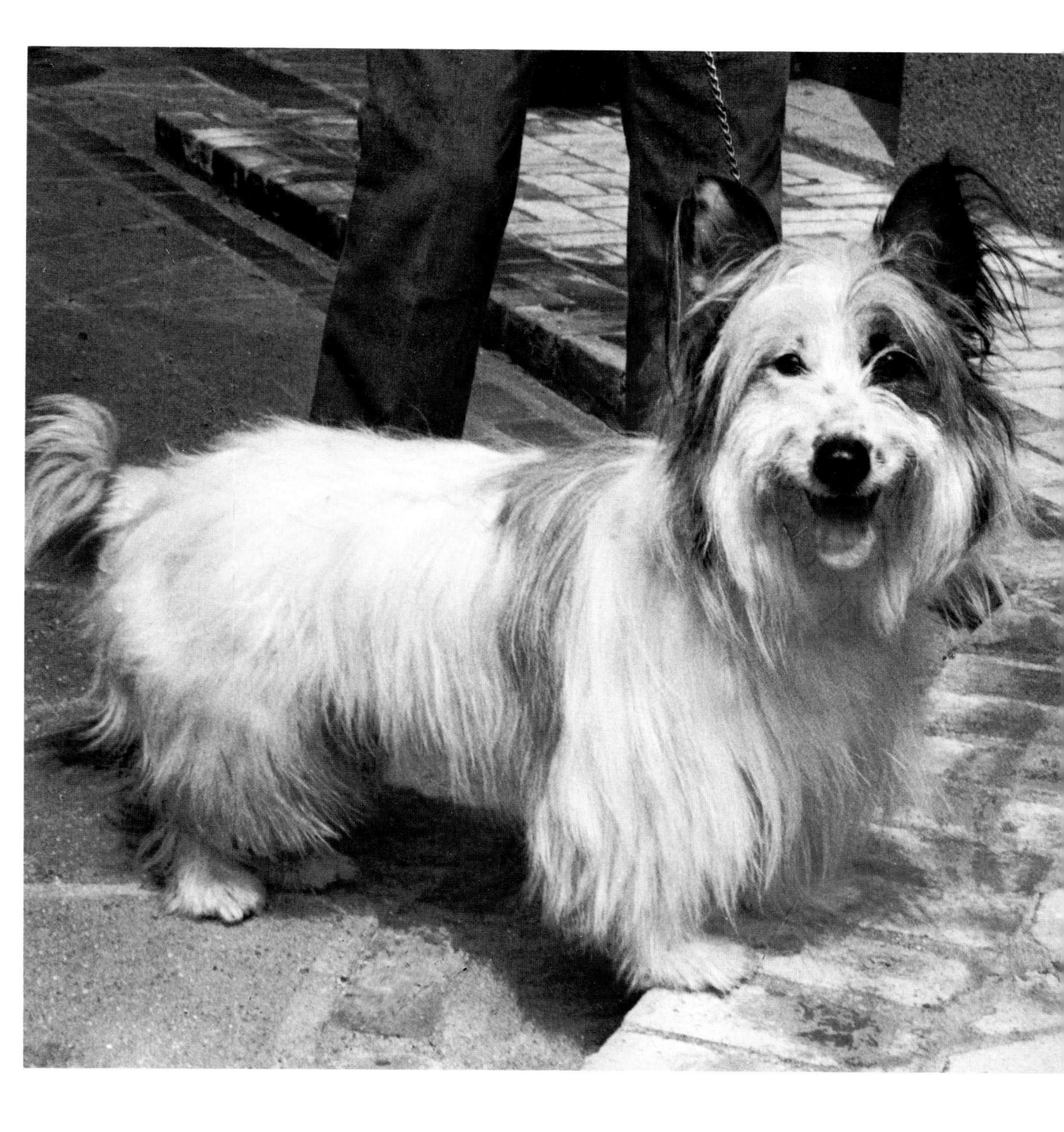

Rascal never knew his parents. His ancestors are a Springer Spaniel and a Wirehaired Dachshund. They are several breeds with white beards, but which was his forefather is not known —it might be the Wirehaired Terrier.

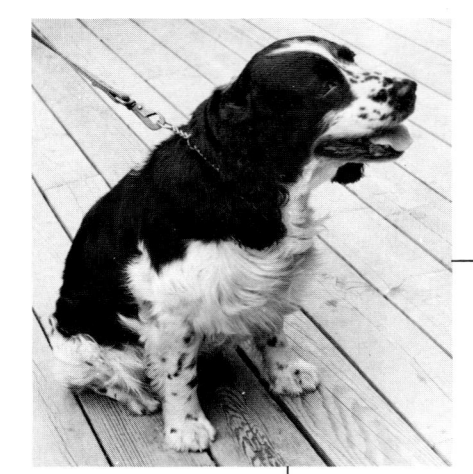

English Springer Spaniel

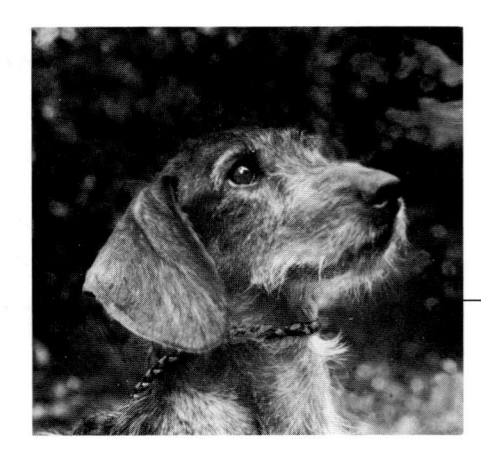

Wirehaired Dachshund

Wirehaired Terrier

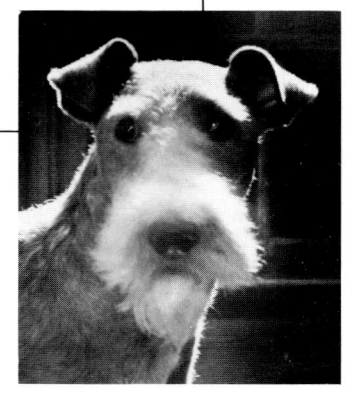

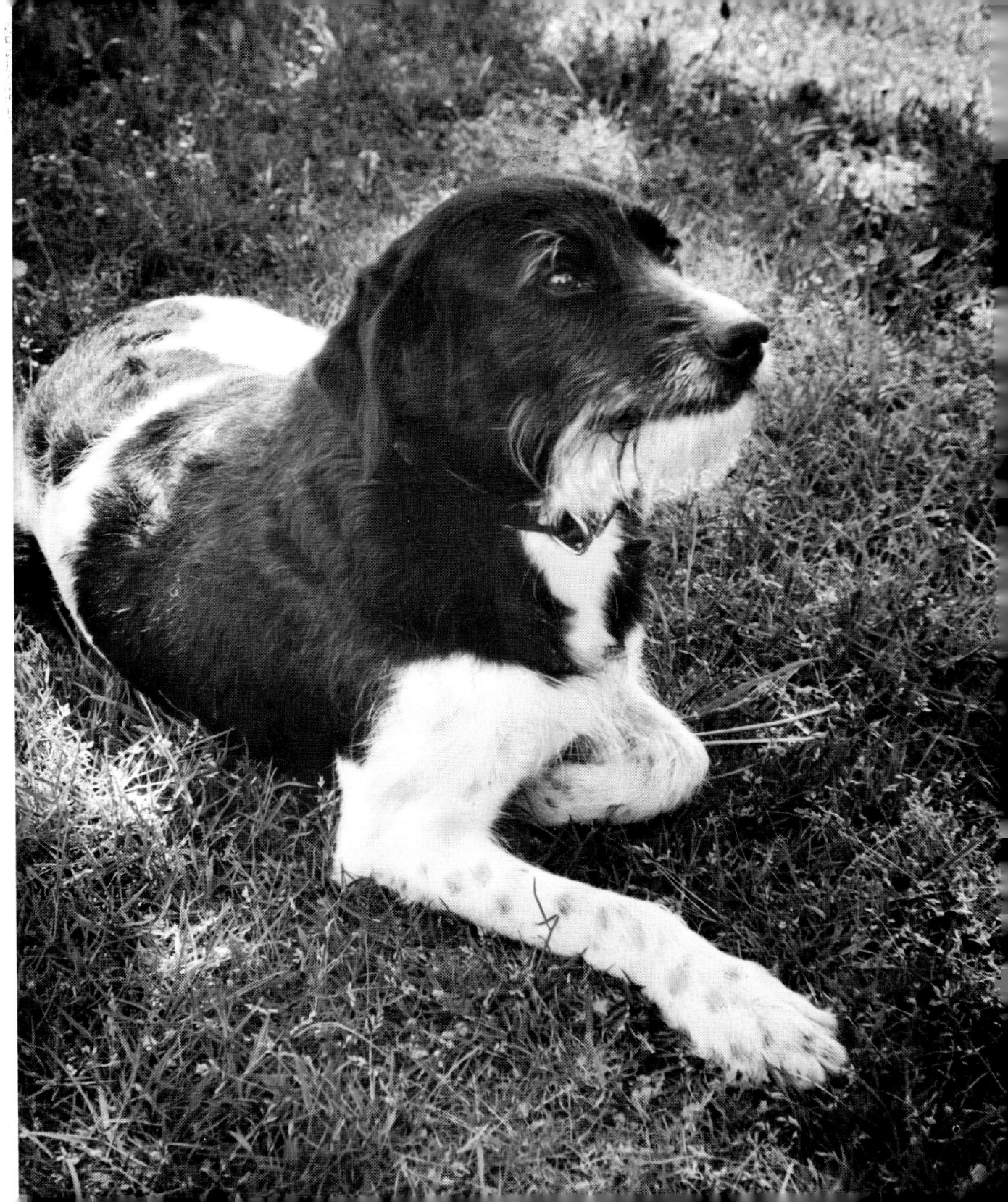

Blondy is not a Cocker Spaniel.
She looks and behaves like a
Cocker Spaniel but she has some
other ancestors too. One of them
is the Poodle. Blondy is not an
accomplished performer, like many
Poodles are, but she is good at
the few tricks she does.
She can "roll over" and jump
a hurdle. It's enough to
impress her public.

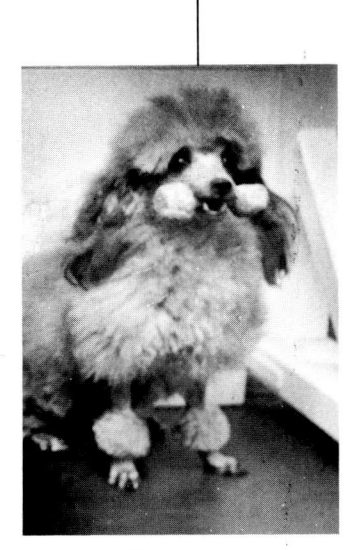

Cocker Spaniel

Poodle

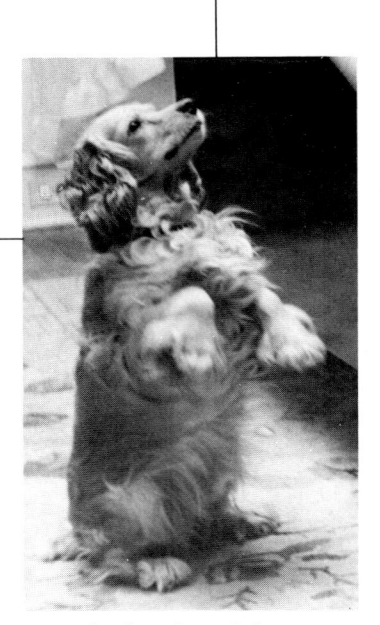

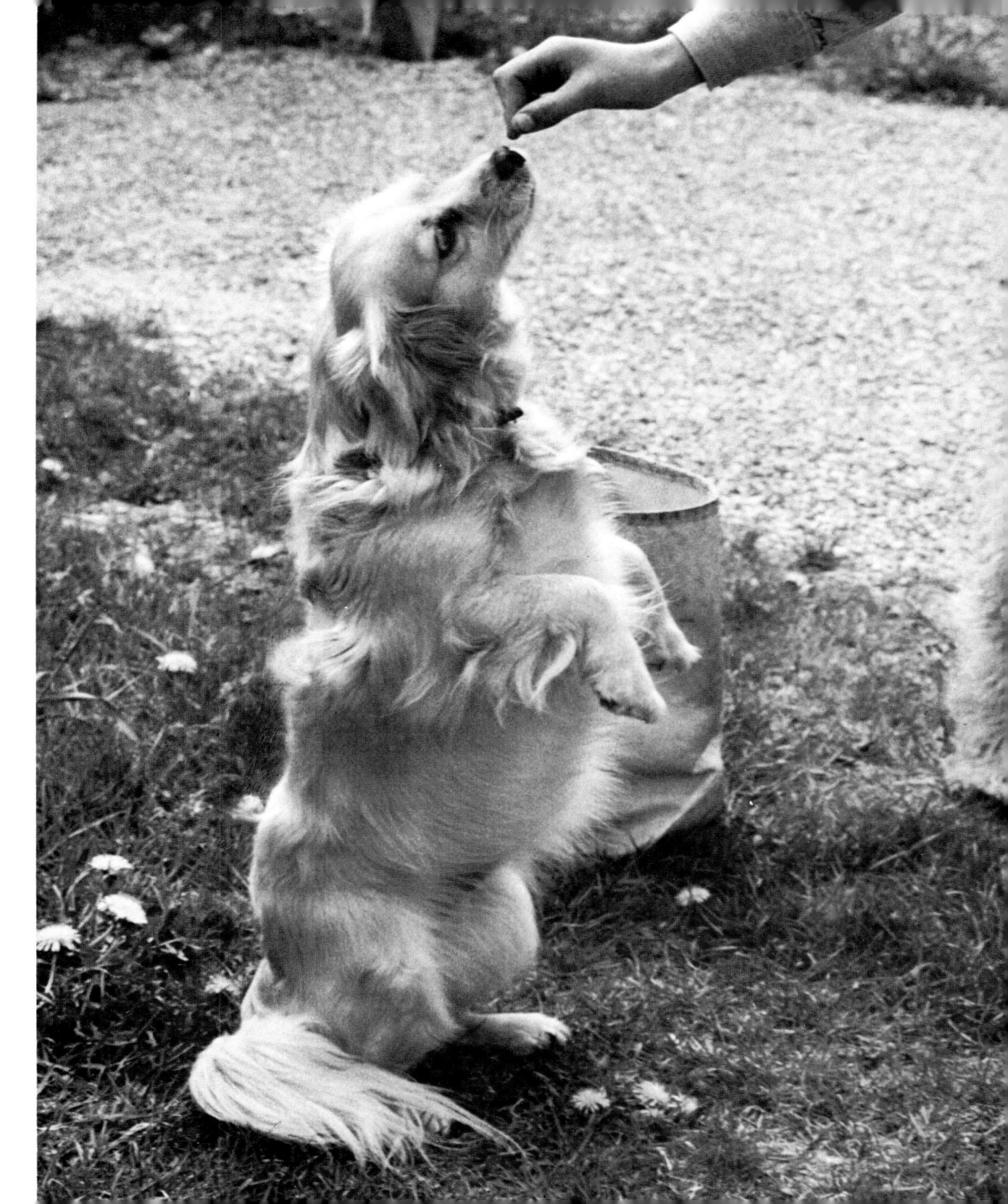

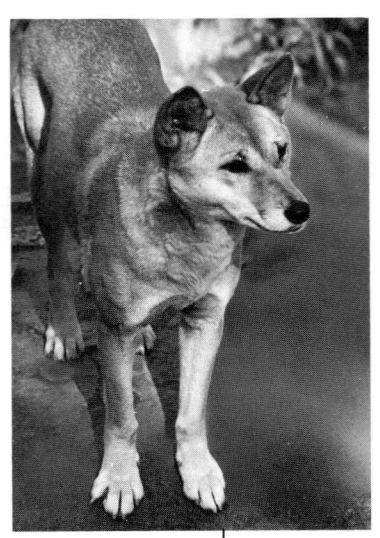

A long way back an Australian Dingo was an ancestor of Bonnie. Sine then many other breeds joined in, including a Collie and a Husky, but the Dingo ancestor is always remembered —a picture of a Dingo hangs on the wall in Bonnie's corner.

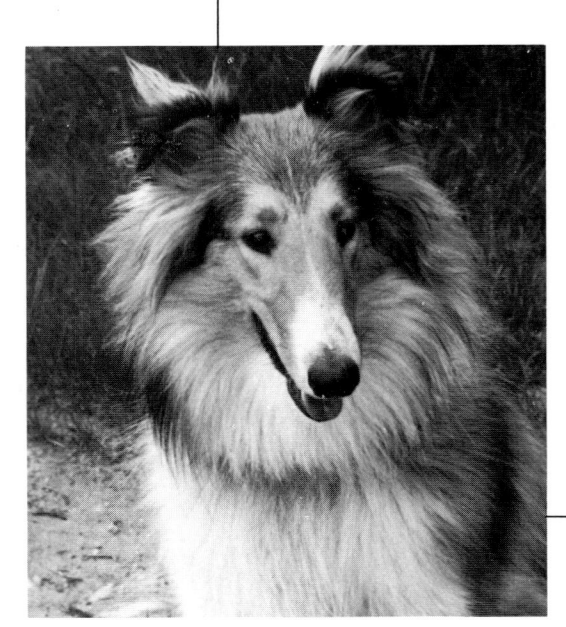

Australian Dingo

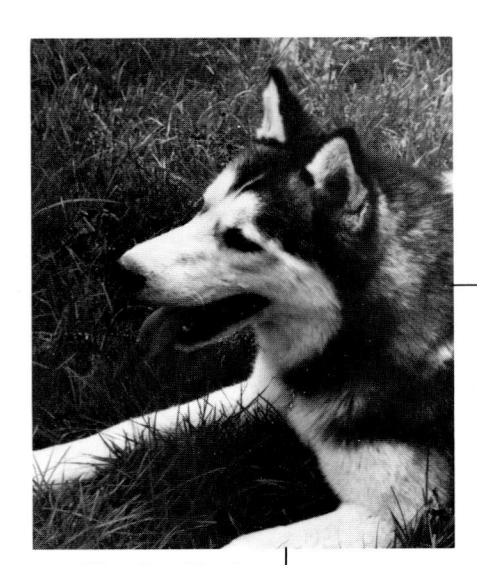

Siberian Husky

Collie

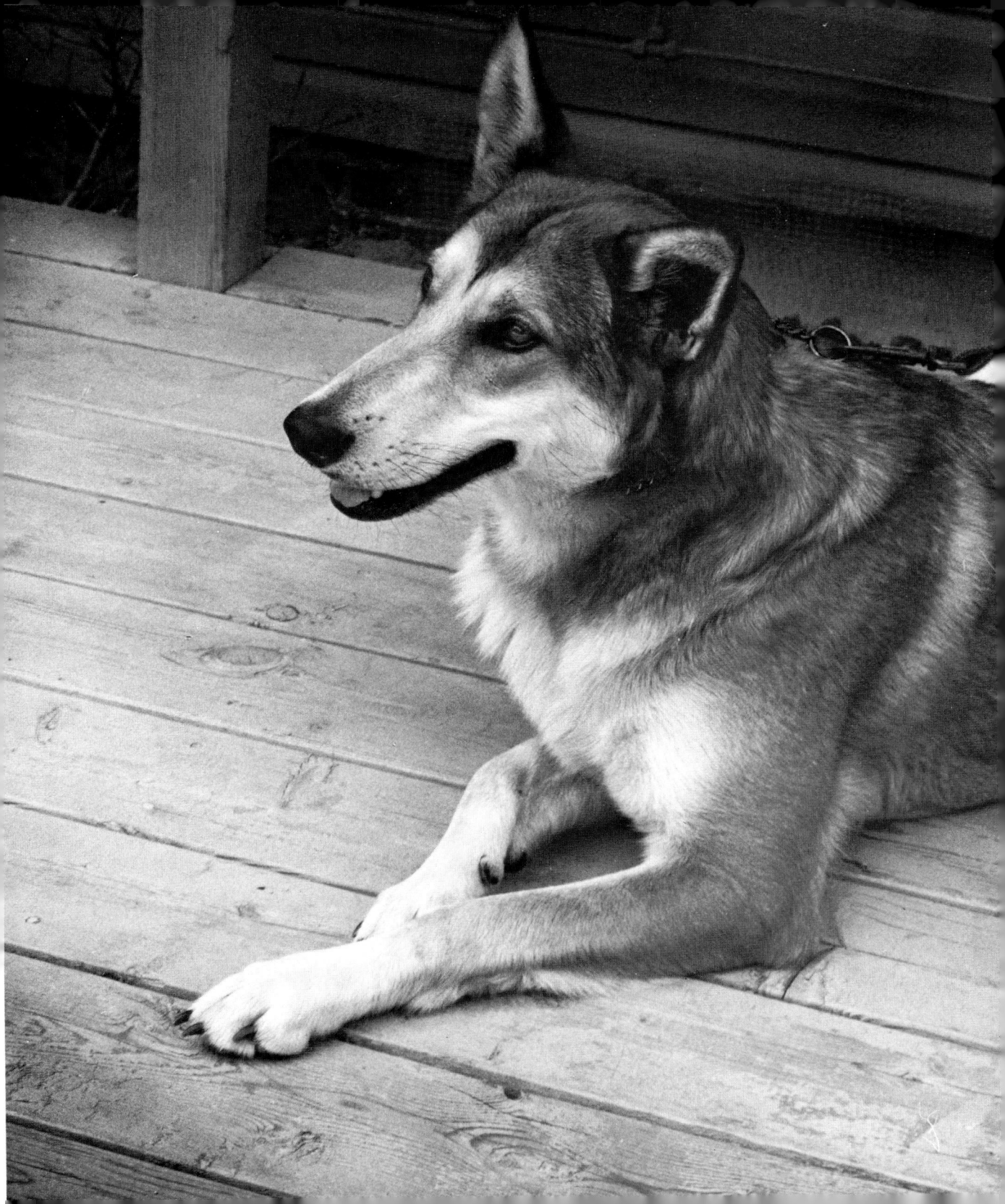

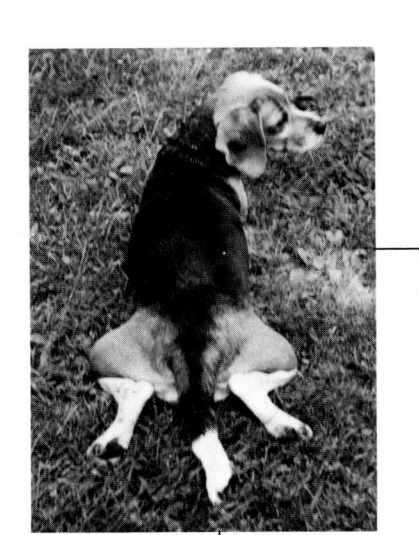

Pepper looks like a composite of Beagle, Basset Hound, and Dachshund. She shares her home with two other dogs, but there is never jealousy or fighting. Pepper does not have a mean bone in her body. Sometimes she looks like a pure-breed—only it is very difficult to pinpoint which one.

Beagle

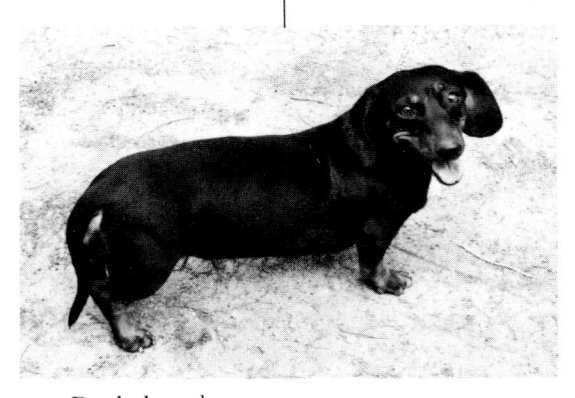

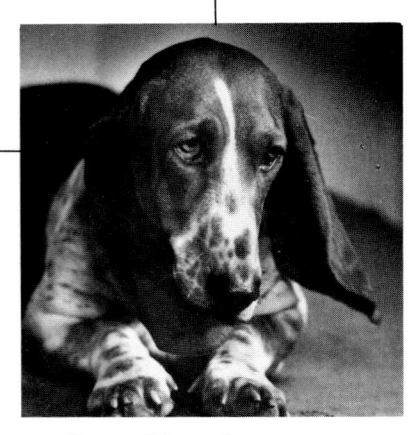

Basset Hound

Dachshund

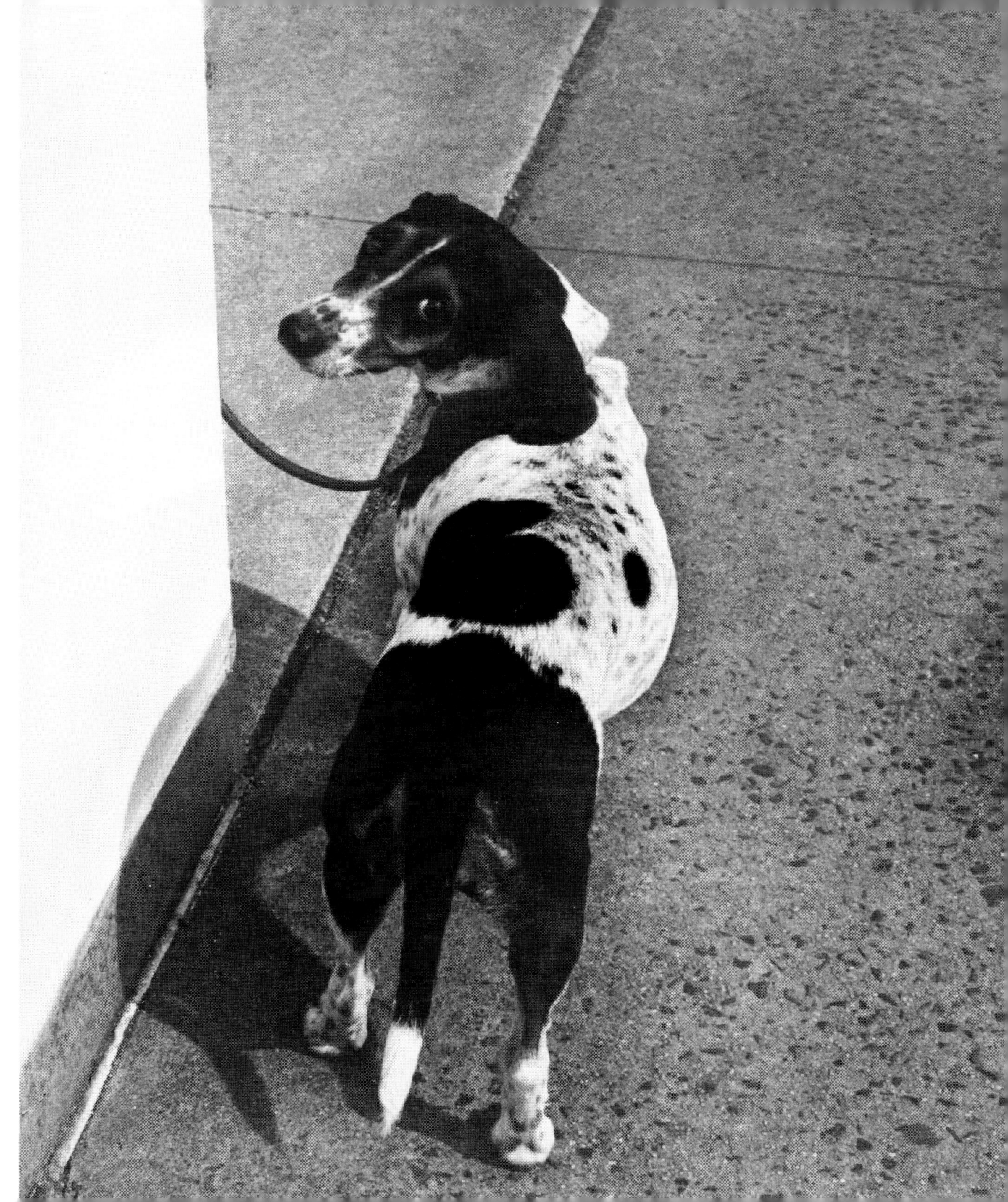

Daisy May is definitely a terrier. She has many terrier breeds in her past parentage, Norwich Terrier, Australian Terrier, and West Highland White Terrier are among them. Her looks vary with haircut and mood —she can look like any one of the breeds, or all combined in one— the new "Daisy May Terrier."

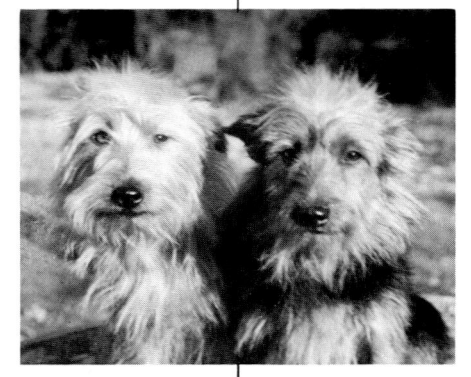

Australian Terriers

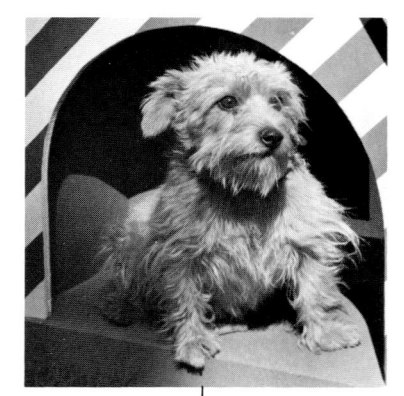

Norwich Terrier

West Highland White Terrier

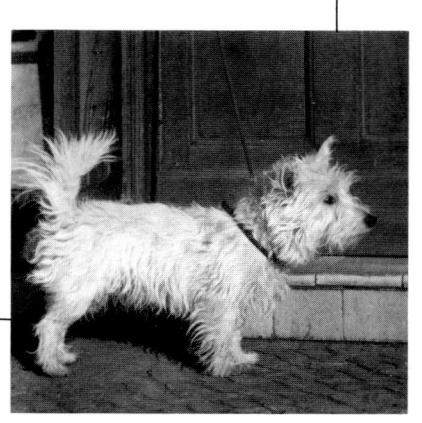

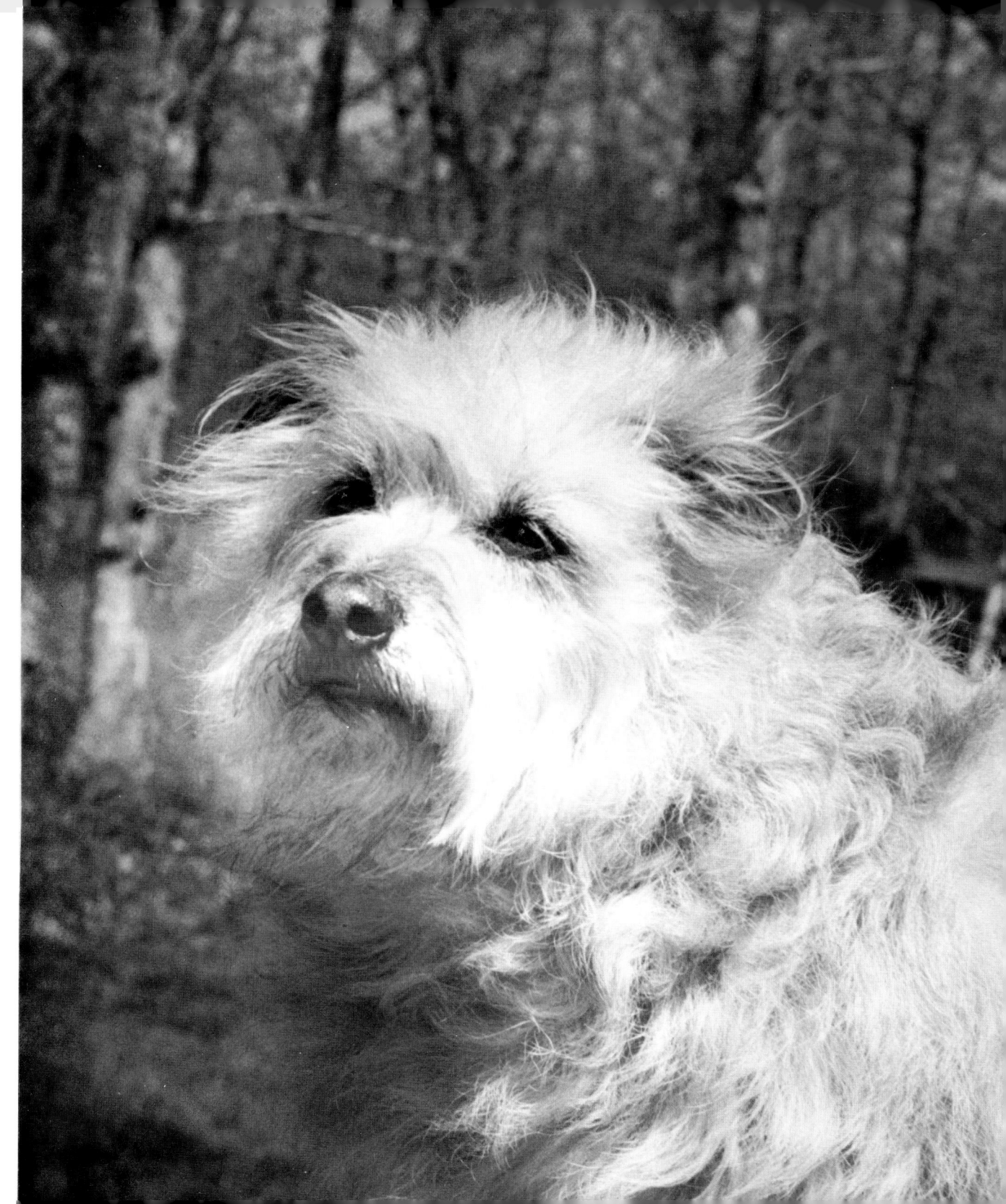

Laverne and Fred are sister and brother. Their parents are a Briard and an Old English Sheepdog. They don't have to herd sheep but they do guard everything else—the grounds, buggy, and family house. To tell them apart, Laverne gets a special haircut.

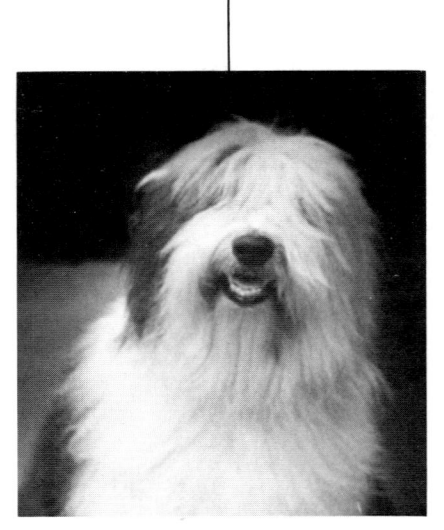

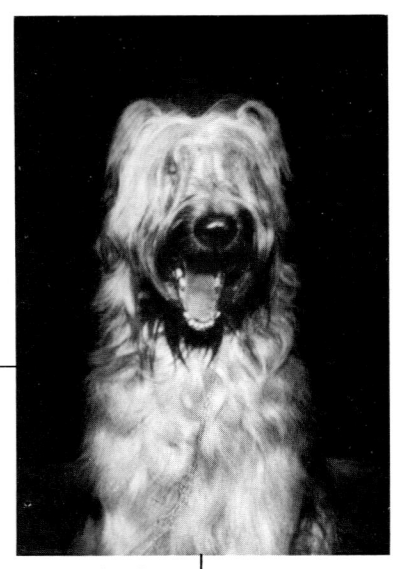

Briard

Old English Sheepdog

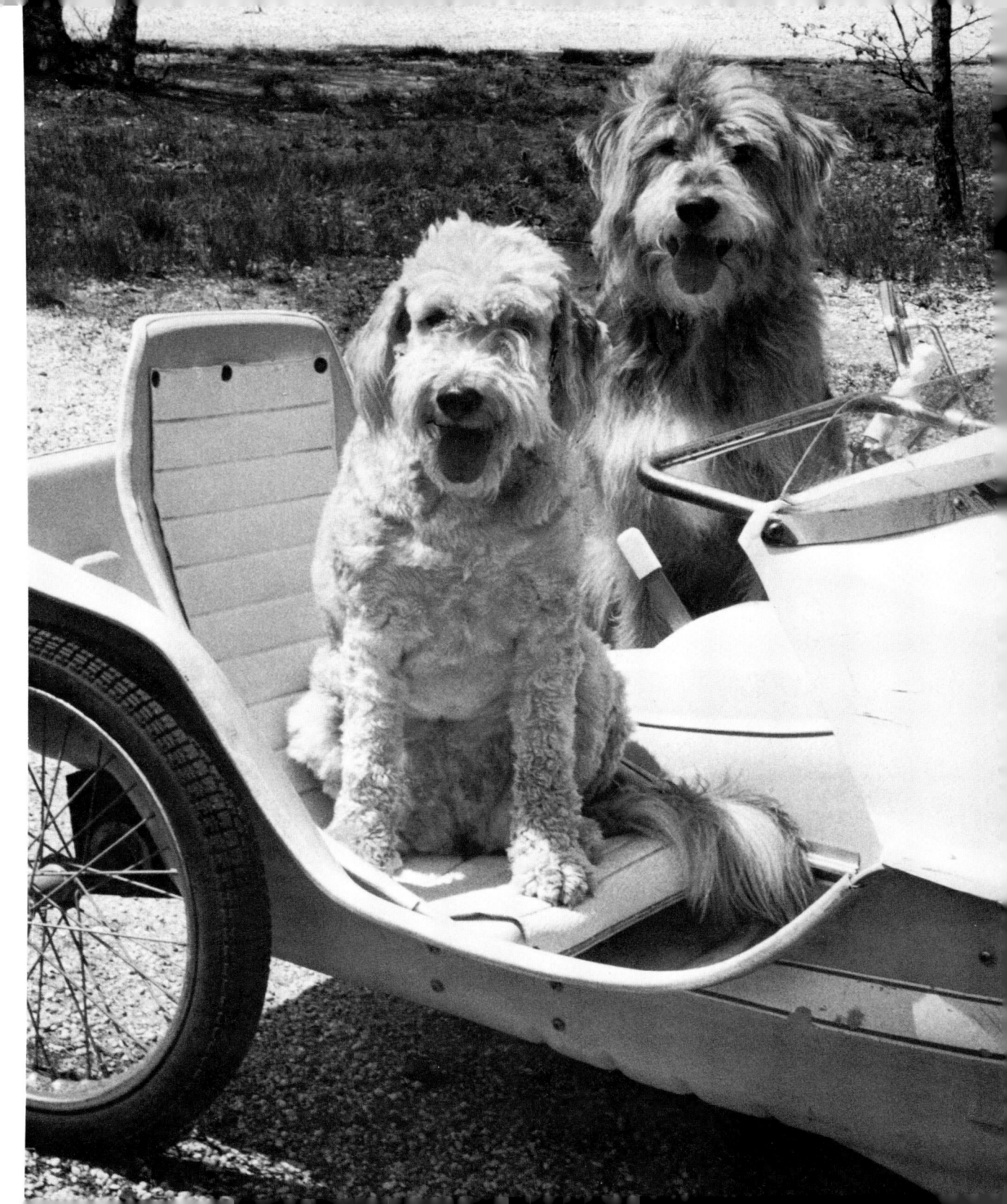

Lady is calm and dignified, she selects her friends very carefully. She dislikes some dogs for no visible reason. Whenever she meets them, she loses her calm and barks. There is speculation about Lady's ancestors: the Black Labrador and Collie have the most votes.

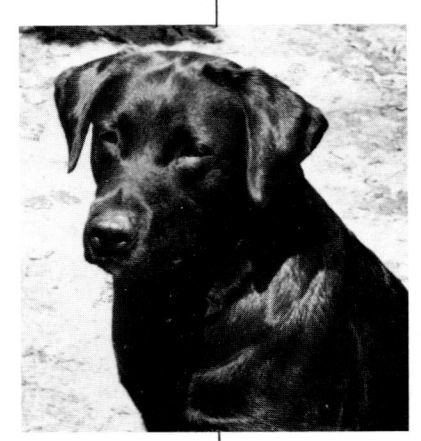

Labrador Retriever

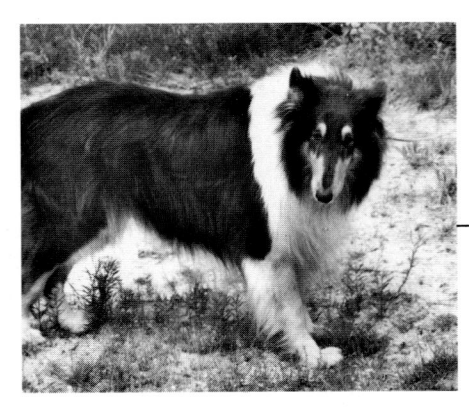

Collie

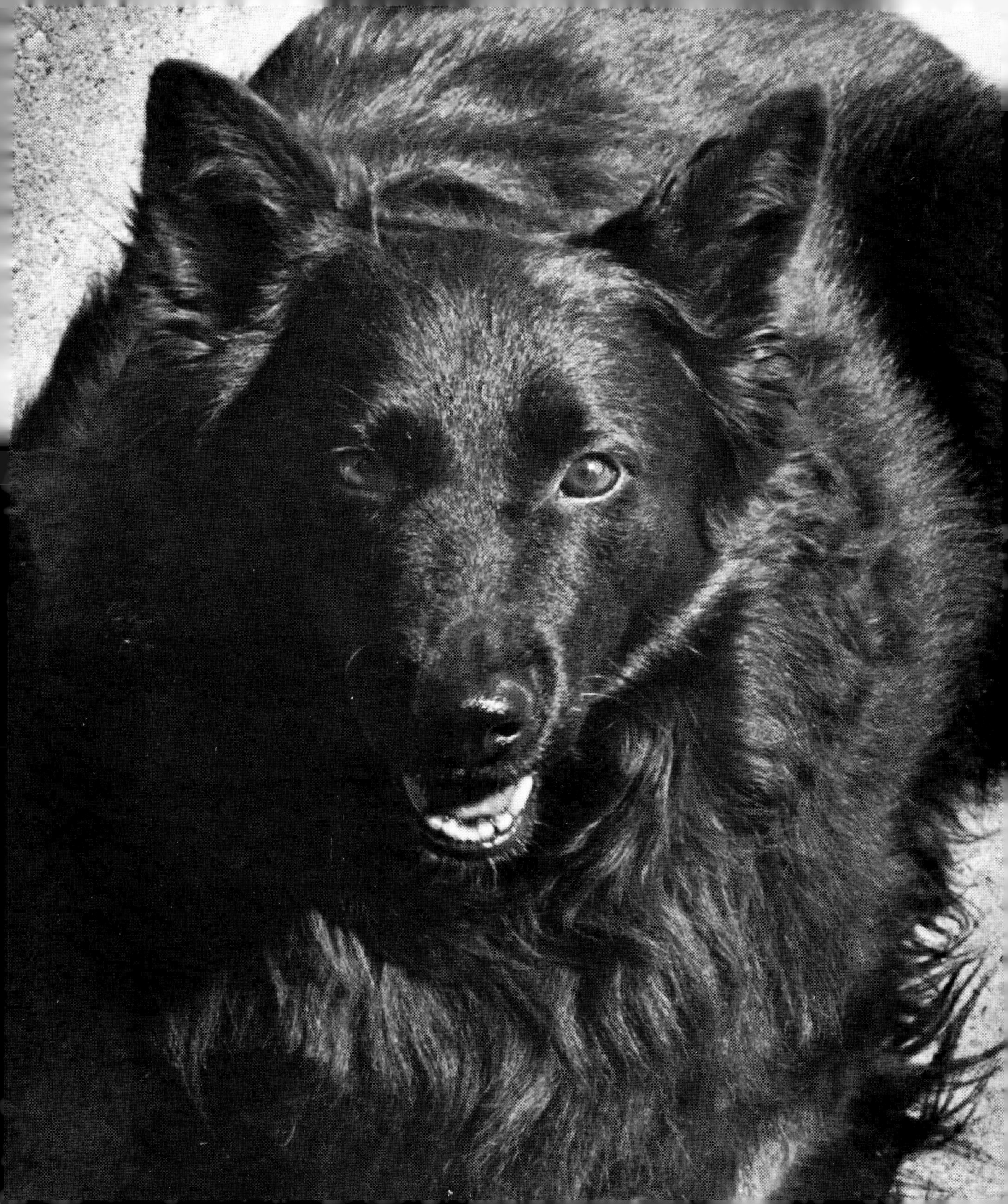

Tuffy's parents are a Schnauzer and a Lhasa Apso. Tuffy spends every weekend on a boat—her favored life-style. She likes to look at the waves but swims only when it's necessary. If the boat leaves without her, she patiently waits at the dock. When the boat returns, Tuffy swims out to meet it.

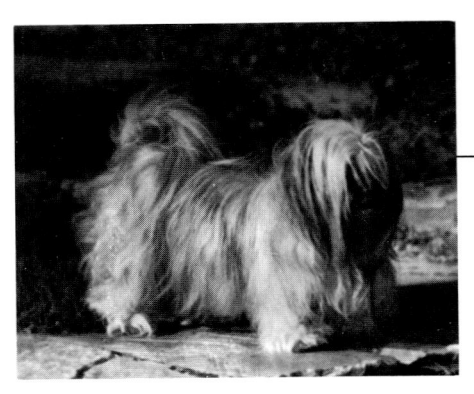

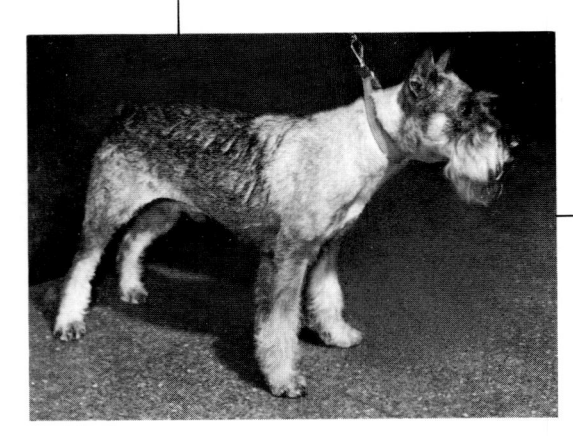

Lhasa Apso

Schnauzer

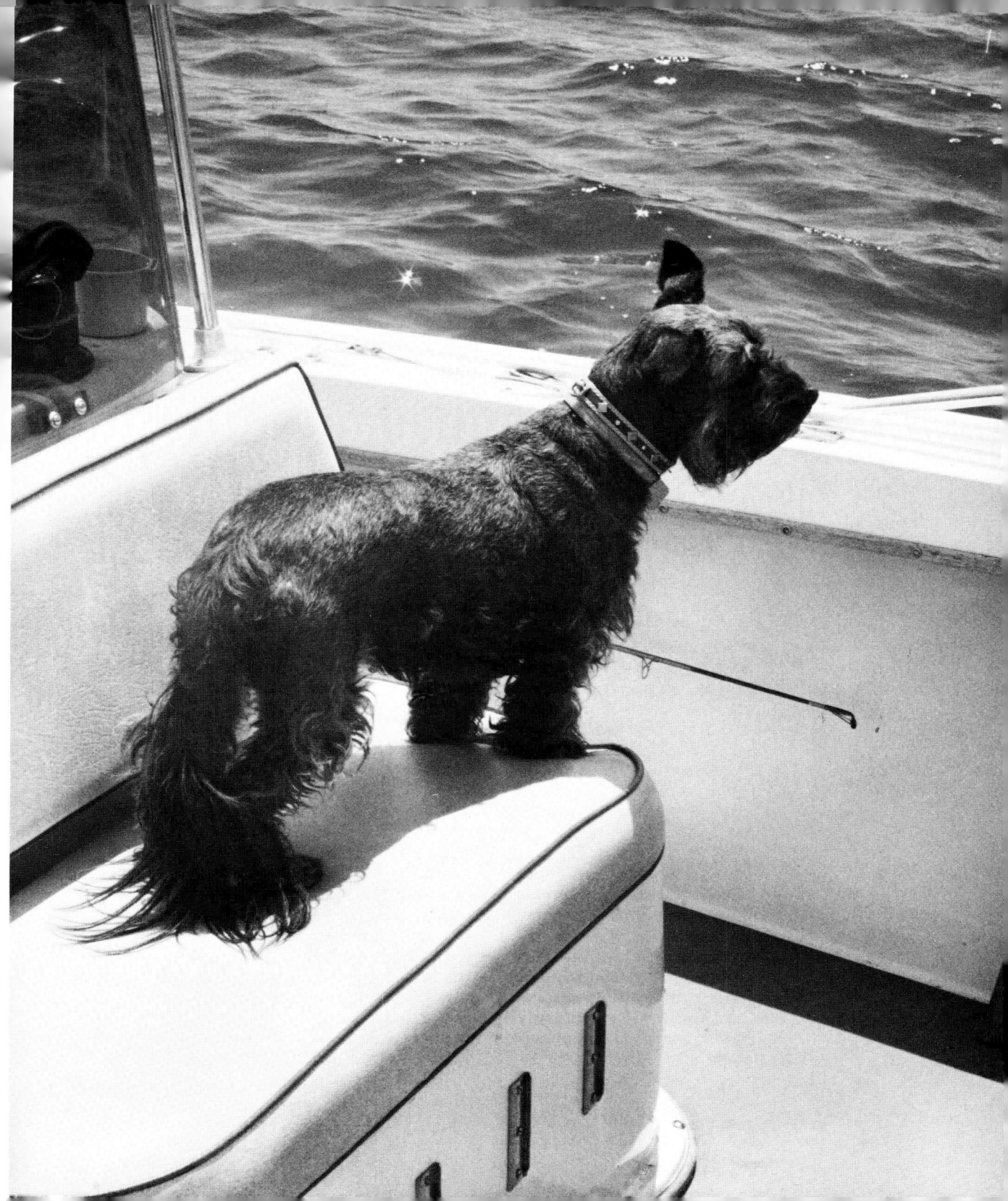

Nobody knows where Ragsy came from. After painful encounters with unfriendly dogs and cars, he now leads a quiet life. He spends most of his time under a bush observing the neighbors. The Norwegian Elkhound was one of his ancestors. When Ragsy's tail is not wagging it's curled over his back. A sure sign of his Chow ancestry is his blue-black tongue. In some Asiatic countries the Chow Chow is raised as a delicacy. Ragsy wouldn't like that.

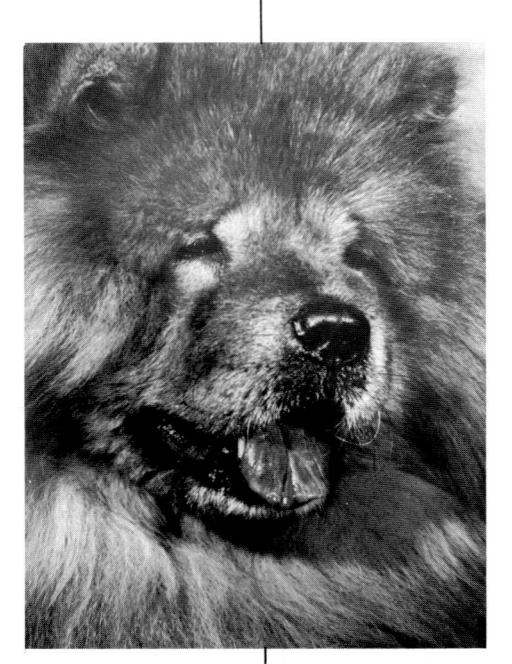

Chow Chow

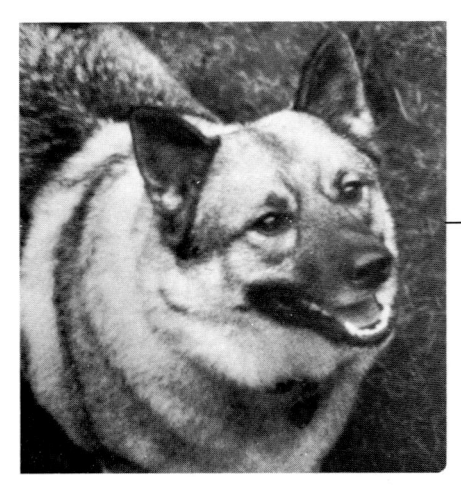

Norwegian Elkhound

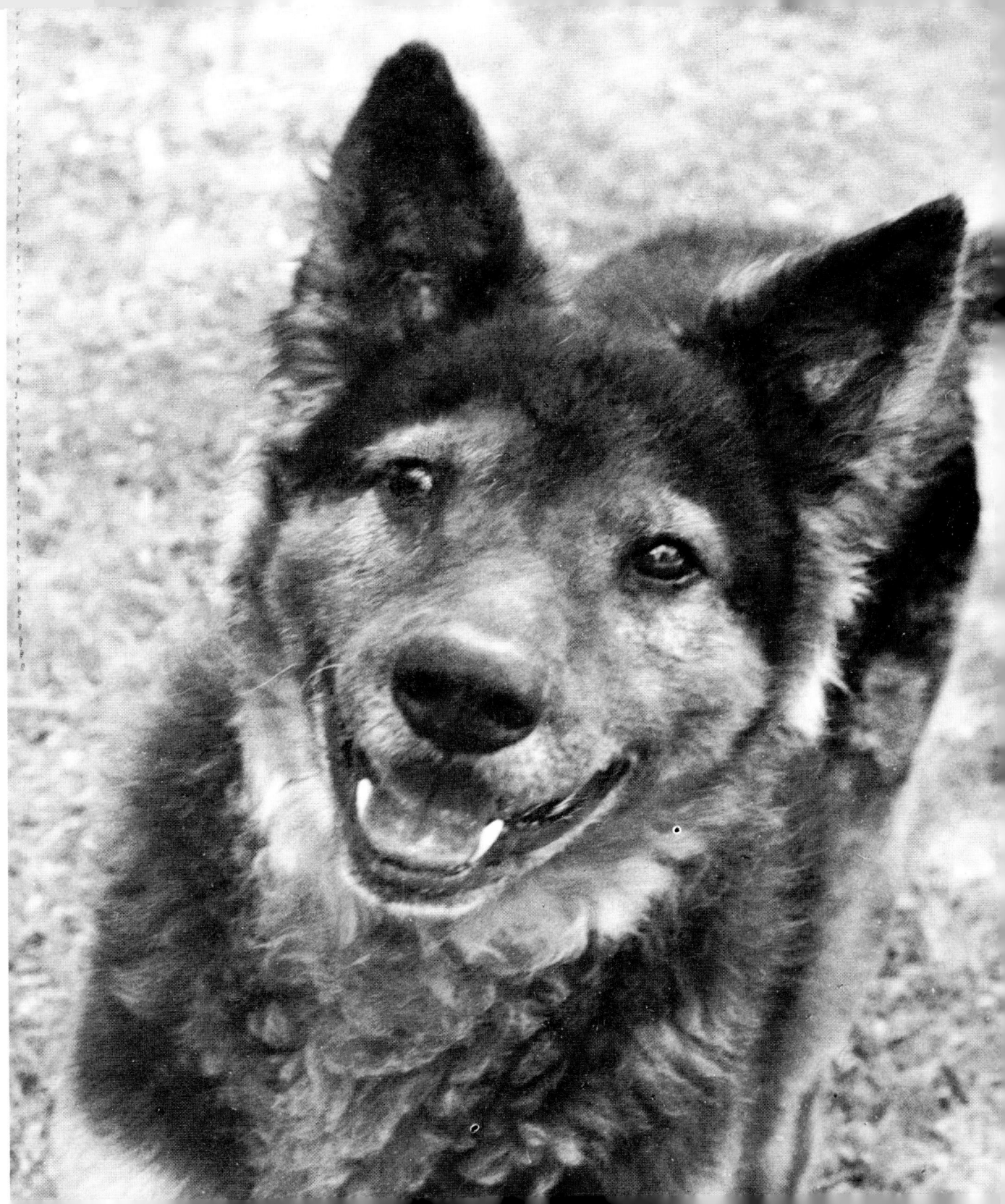

For many months, Lundy was walking through city streets looking for food and shelter. She was lost or abandoned. One day, abused, tired, hungry, and weak, she found a home in the city with a place in the country, where she can play and run. In the opinion of experts, she is a mix of Belgian Tervueren and Collie. Lundy doesn't care about her ancestors—she is happy now.

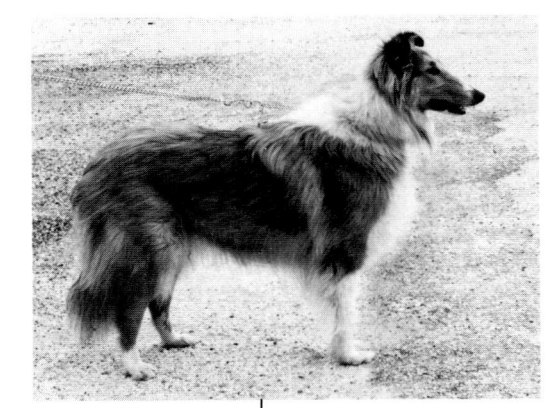

Collie

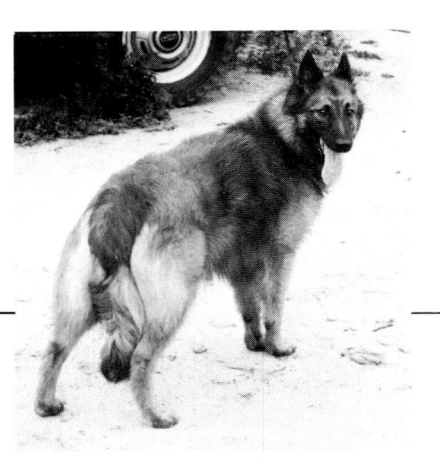

Belgian Tervueren Shepherd

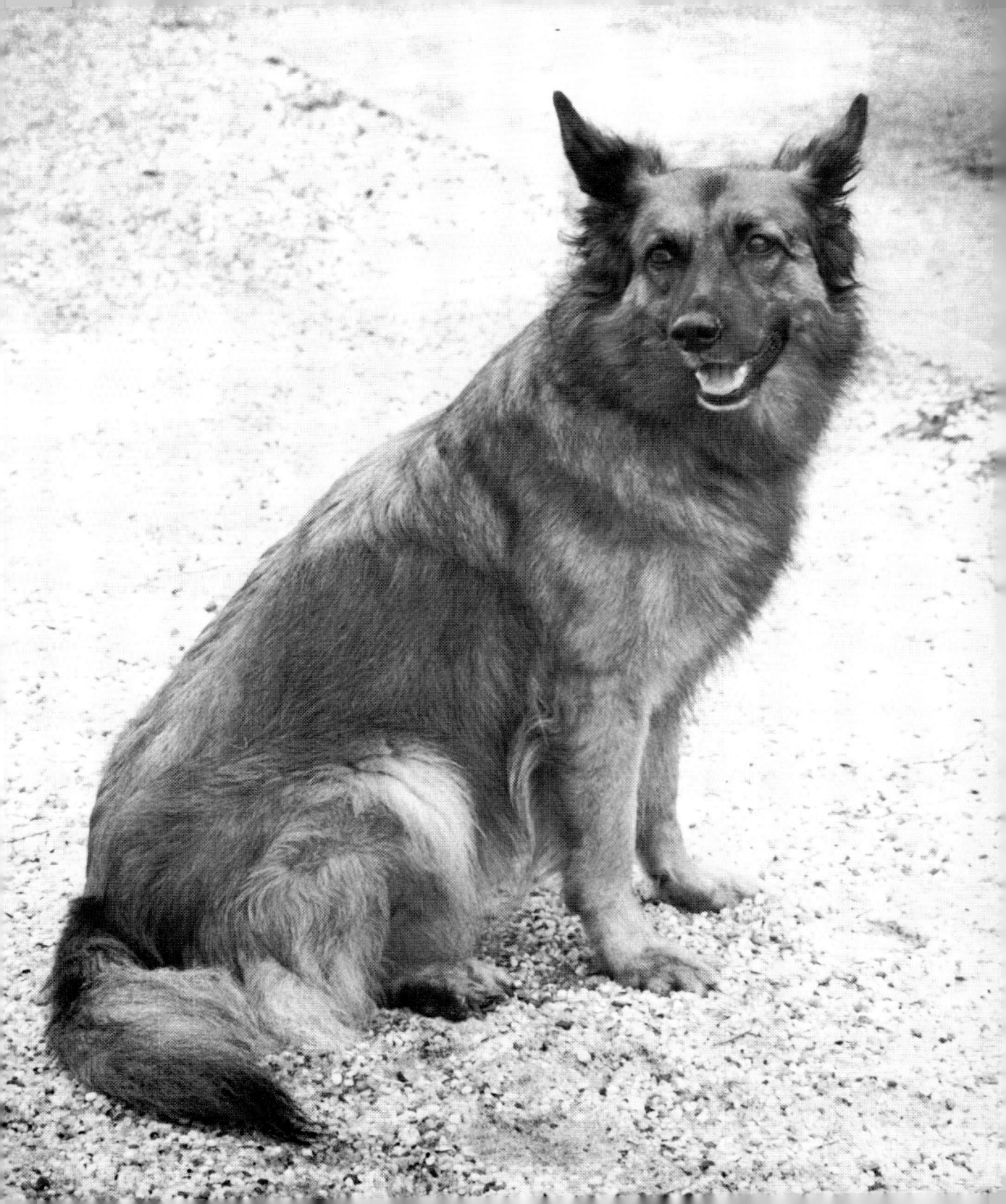

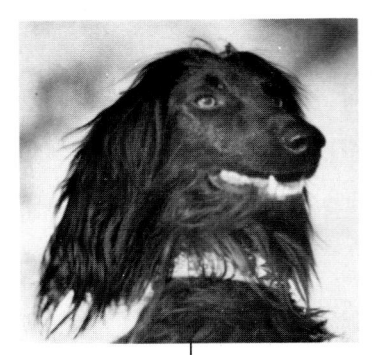

Afghan Hound

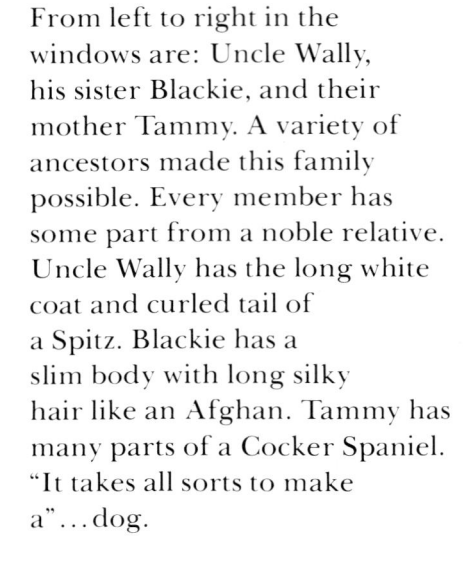

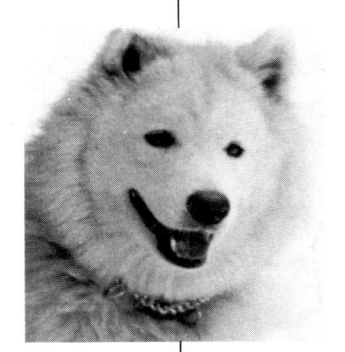

Spitz

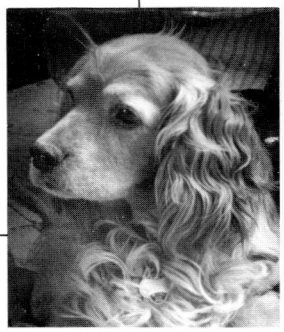

Cocker Spaniel

From left to right in the windows are: Uncle Wally, his sister Blackie, and their mother Tammy. A variety of ancestors made this family possible. Every member has some part from a noble relative. Uncle Wally has the long white coat and curled tail of a Spitz. Blackie has a slim body with long silky hair like an Afghan. Tammy has many parts of a Cocker Spaniel. "It takes all sorts to make a"...dog.

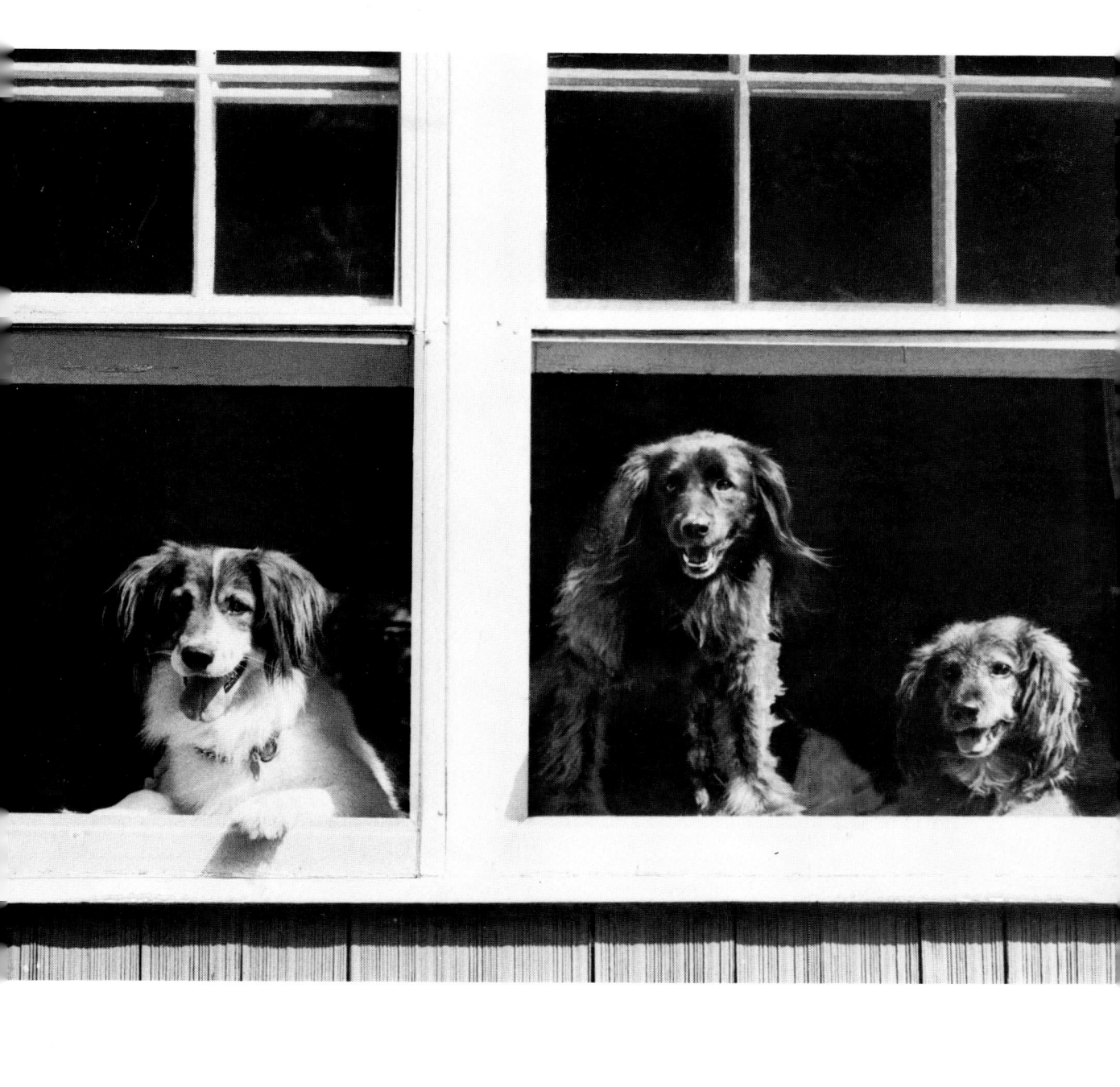

Many breeds, often unfamiliar to the average dog-owner, could be in the ancestry of a mongrel; here are some of them.

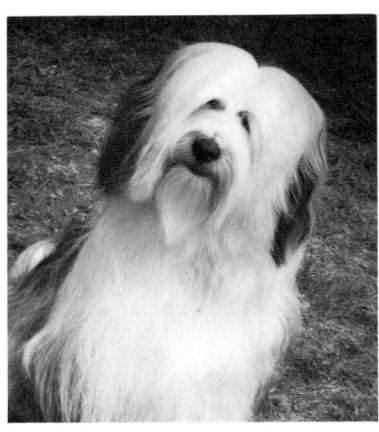

The Tibetan Terrier comes from a remote region. The little dog is a highly valuable herder in the mountains of Tibet.

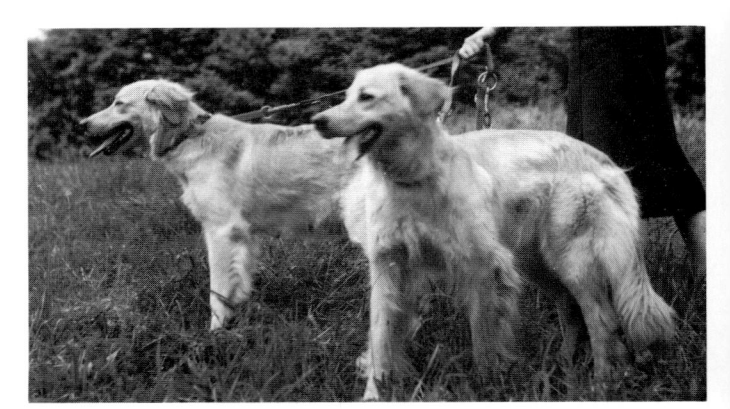

Hovawarts are a new German breed, with ancestors traced back to the first European shepherd dog—the Bronze Age Dog.

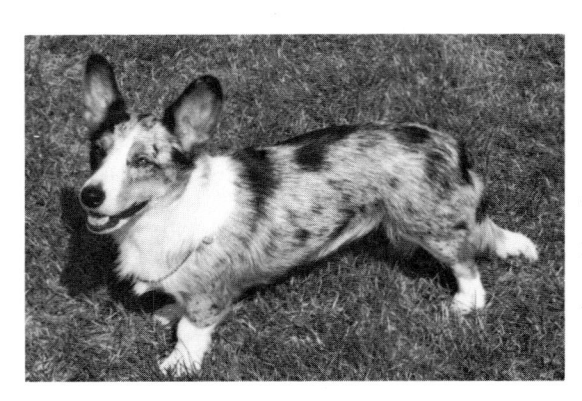

The Cardigan Welsh Corgi is often marked merle: his coat is covered with blue, white, gray, and black spots.

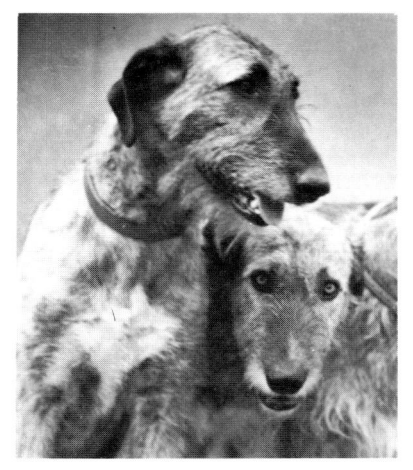

Irish Wolfhounds are the largest dogs in the world. Few people know how gentle and devoted these powerful giants are.

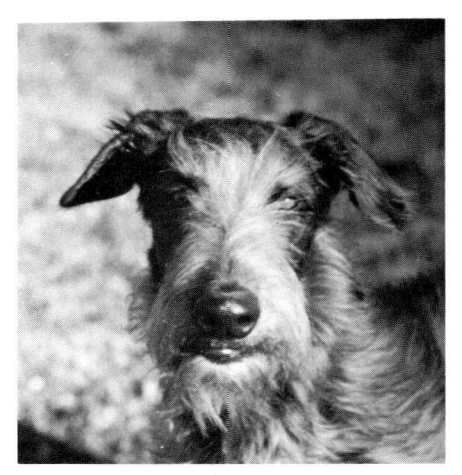

The Scottish Deerhound was known as "The Royal Dog of Scotland." In past centuries only noblemen could own the Deerhound.

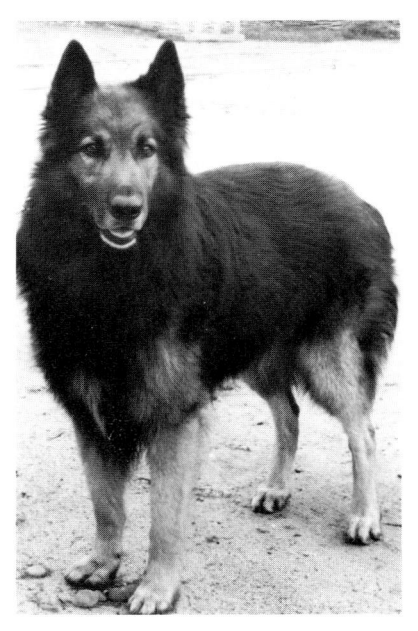

The Tervueren is a Belgian Sheepdog. The male has a dark coat, the female is tawny-gold.

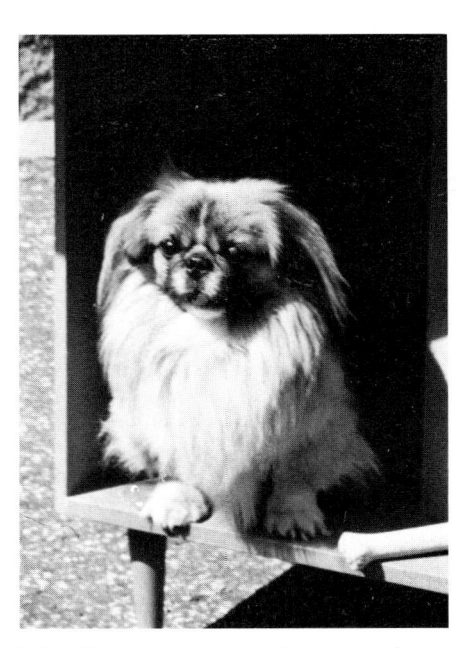

The Pekingese was the sacred palace dog in Peking, China. This little dog is fearless, dignified, strong, and totally devoted to its owner.

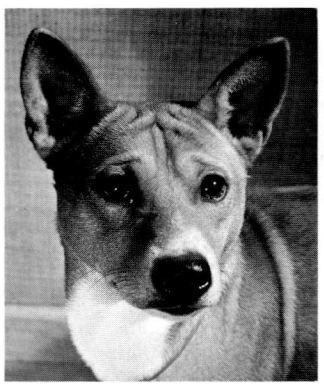

The Basenji is the barkless dog of Africa. He has a glossy coat which he cleans like a cat. The wrinkles on his forehead give him a thoughtful expression.

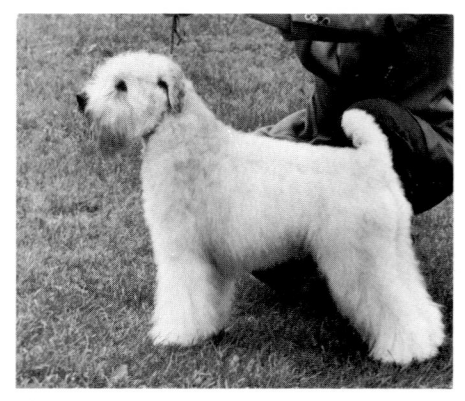

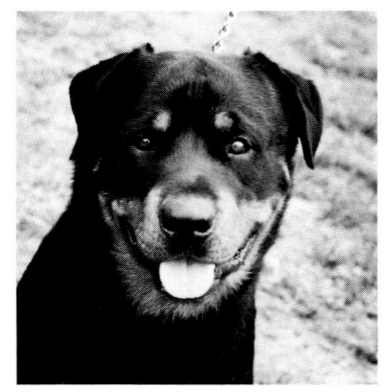

The Rottweiler is a courageous guard dog. He is a descendant of the Roman cattle dogs.

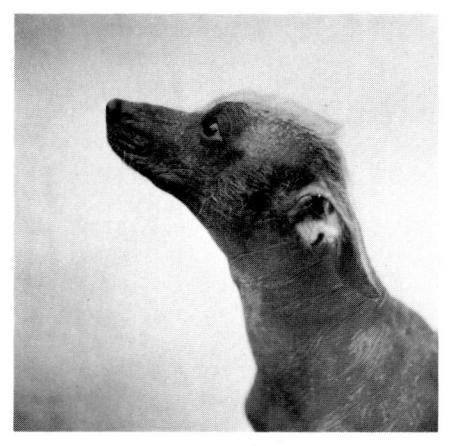

The Soft-coated Wheaten Terrier is an Irish breed with a thick weather-resistant coat. He is robust, agile, and very affectionate.

The African Hairless is soft and warm. He is a "living barometer," his skin is light gray when the weather is fair; it changes to dull dark when the weather gets bad.

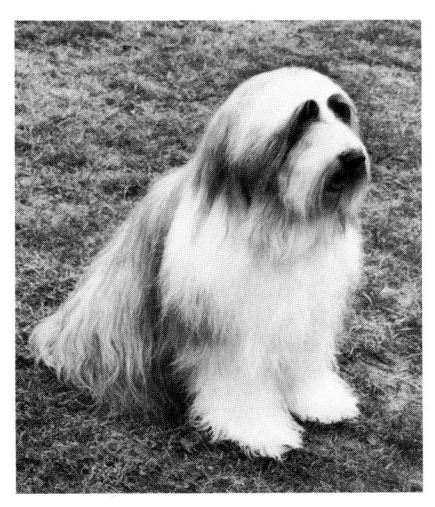

The Bearded Collie has the appealing look of a large toy. In old times he was a sheepdog, now he is an active, friendly pet.

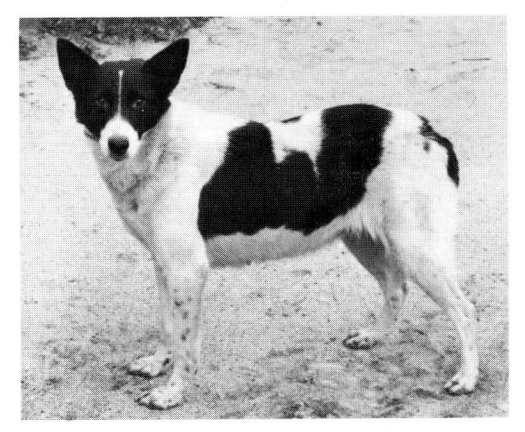

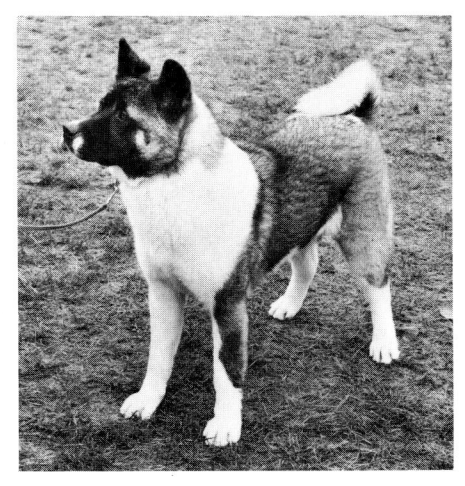

The Akita is the national Japanese dog. A member of the Spitz family, the Akita has most unusual markings.

The Canaan Dog originated in the Land of Canaan, over 3,000 years ago. For many years they lived wild in the Negev Desert. Now redomesticated by the Israelis, these dogs have proved to be highly intelligent and easy to train.

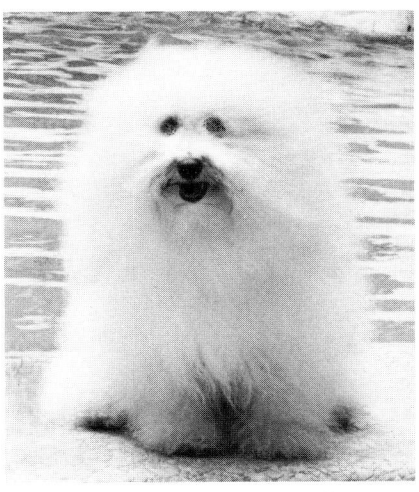

The Bichon Frise looks like a living "powder puff," but this little dog is sturdy, playful, and likes to swim.